Disease and Its Control

Disease and Its Control

THE SHAPING OF MODERN THOUGHT

Robert P. Hudson

PRAEGER

New York
Westport, Connecticut
London

Library of Congress Cataloging-in-Publication Data

Hudson, Robert P.
  Disease and its control.

  Includes bibliographies and index.
    1. Medicine—History. 2. Medicine—Philosophy.
  I. Title.
  [R131.H825 1987]   616'.009   87-9340
  ISBN 0-275-92779-2 (pbk. : alk. paper)

A hardcover edition of *Disease and Its Control: The Shaping of Modern Thought*
is available from Greenwood Press (Contributions in Medical Studies; 12;
ISBN 0-313-23806-5).

Library of Congress Catalog Card Number: 87-9340
ISBN: 0-275-92779-2

First published 1983

Paperback edition 1987

Praeger Publishers, One Madison Avenue, New York, NY 10010
A division of Greenwood Press, Inc.

Printed in the United States of America

The paper used in this book complies with the Permanent
Paper Standard issued by the National
Information Standards Organization (Z39.48-1984).

P

For Jean who made it possible
and
Martha who made it worthwhile

CONTENTS

PREFACE

This book is intended for anyone making an early encounter with the development of medical thinking about the nature of disease and its control. It will be helpful as well to students and teachers whose emphasis in training has been on social or technological aspects of medical history, and to general historians whose goals direct them into the realm of disease.

The history of medicine can be written from several points of view. The biographical path leads one through the lives and contributions of individuals in the history of medicine, the emphasis on "great doctors" which dominated medical history in the past. The social approach emphasizes the interplay between medicine and other social institutions, the manner in which medicine shapes and is shaped by society. The technical history of medicine stresses discovery in the basic sciences and considers the history of medicine as a chapter in the history of biology and technology. The aim of this book is to examine the major concepts that led to our present understanding of disease and its control in the West.

Such divisions of historical labor, of course, are ultimately artificial. Concepts of disease are not freestanding intellectual constructs. They develop in the minds of "great doctors" and others, who in turn are influenced by prevailing social and cultural forces, the available technological resources, and the contemporary level of understanding of physiology and pathology. Ideally, medical history would be a balanced blend of all these approaches, and such a global track is possible for individual diseases, but not in a short, general survey of concepts of disease as they have developed over the entire span of the written word.

Utilizing major concepts as chapter headings could convey the impression that the present effort is a collection of more or less unrelated essays. Nothing could have been further from my intent. In reality the various concepts considered were interlocked throughout their history, though to various degrees depending on time and place. Apparently contradictory conceptions coexisted at times, as do notions of disease as natural and supernatural on the present scene. The ascendancy of one concept had profound effects on others, as the germ theory did on ideas of prevention and treatment. A single concept, the anatomical idea, has had an uninterrupted existence since it assumed importance in medical thinking of the Renaissance, thereafter influencing physiology, pathology, physical diagnosis, and practically every aspect of specificity of disease and its control characterizing current medical thought.

Diseases are not immutable entities but dynamic social constructions that have biographies of their own. Many human conditions which were defined as diseases in past years are no longer recognized, just as most of the terms denoting diseases nowadays would have been alien to earlier medical lexicons. On numerous occasions diseases come into being as a result of social forces not related directly to medical science. If a medical and social consensus defined freckles as a disease, this benign and often winsome skin condition would become a disease. Patients would consult physicians complaining of freckles, physicians would diagnose and treat freckles, and presumably, in time we would have a National Institute of Freckle Research. The concept of disease as mutable is one of the more important ideas in the history of medicine, and one often accepted reluctantly by health professionals themselves.

Western conceptions of disease begin with the notion of disease as supernatural and end with our present perception of diseases as natural, specific, and associated with specific causes. A central theme in this story is the shift from disease as generalized to disease as localized in its origins. This crucial change in outlook resulted from the anatomical idea, or the anatomical way of thinking. The spread of this new orientation led to an improved understanding of physiology and ultimately to the notion that disease originated within localized structures of the body. Ever increasingly sophisticated practices of experimental medicine, particularly in the nineteenth century, culminated in the germ theory of disease, or for our purposes, the belief that specific diseases have specific causes. Since our conceptions of causation often dictate the nature of actions taken to control disease, the story would not be complete without a survey of preventive medicine and therapy.

Finally, the evolution of thought about disease can be viewed by making a distinction between disease and illness. At various times diseases have been seen as having an existence of their own (the ontological view), and at other times they have been held to be unique episodes or illnesses in single individuals over time (the physiological conception). Both ways of looking at disease have deficiencies and merits. The present tendency is to avoid one-sided thinking and to meld both ideas into a single approach to medical education and practice. The student perforce studies disease, but the wise practitioner uses his knowledge of disease to treat and prevent illness. Such are the themes explored in what follows.

ACKNOWLEDGMENTS

I benefited greatly from a number of critical readings of this manuscript, most notably those by John T. Alexander, Gert H. Brieger, Frederic L. Holmes, and Robert Joy. At the same time I hasten to exonerate them from the ultimate fate of their suggestions. I am grateful as well to John Burnham for his excellent editorial guidance during the later revisions of the manuscript.

There is no way I can compensate Lena Downing for her faithful and superb typing of the manuscript "one more time." Thanks also to Bernice Dean Jackson and others in the Clendening Library for treating each of my routine requests as though it was urgent.

Finally, I am indebted to my wife Martha for her moral support and critical eye and to Stephen and Laurel for staying away from the study door as best they could.

ABBREVIATIONS
OF JOURNALS

Am. Anthropologist	*American Anthropologist*
Am. Hist. Rev.	*American Historical Review*
Am. J. Phys. Anthropol.	*American Journal of Physical Anthropology*
Ann. Int. Med.	*Annals of Internal Medicine*
Ann. Med. Hist.	*Annals of Medical History*
Arch. Gen. Psychiat.	*Archives of General Psychiatry*
Brit. Med. J.	*British Medical Journal*
Bull. Am. Soc. Hosp. Pharm.	*Bulletin of the American Society of Hospital Pharmacists*
Bull. Hist. Med.	*Bulletin of the History of Medicine*
Bull. Inst. Hist. Med.	*Bulletin of the Institute of the History of Medicine*
Bull. Johns Hopkins Hosp.	*Bulletin of the Johns Hopkins Hospital*
Bull. N.Y. Acad. Med.	*Bulletin of the New York Academy of Medicine*
Glasgow Med. J.	*Glasgow Medical Journal*
Hist. Sci.	*History of Science*

Interstate Med. J.	*Interstate Medical Journal*
J. Am. Med. Assn.	*Journal of the American Medical Association*
J. Am. Hist.	*Journal of American History*
J. Brit. Studies	*Journal of British Studies*
J. Chronic Diseases	*Journal of Chronic Diseases*
J. Hellenistic Studies	*Journal of Hellenistic Studies*
J. Hist. Behav. Sci.	*Journal of the History of the Behavioral Sciences*
J. Hist. Ideas	*Journal of the History of Ideas*
J. Hist. Med. and Allied Sciences	*Journal of the History of Medicine and Allied Sciences*
J. Mental Sci.	*Journal of Mental Science*
Johns Hopkins Hosp. Bull.	*Johns Hopkins Hospital Bulletin*
J. Roy. Soc. Med.	*Journal of the Royal Society of Medicine*
Med. Hist.	*Medical History*
New Eng. J. Med.	*New England Journal of Medicine*
Perspectives Bio. and Med.	*Perspectives in Biology and Medicine*
Phil. and Public Affairs	*Philosophy and Public Affairs*
Phil. Sci.	*Philosophy of Science*
Proc. Roy. Soc. Med.	*Proceedings of The Royal Society of Medicine*
Roy. Soc. Health J.	*Royal Society Health Journal*
Sci., Med., and Man	*Science, Medicine and Man*
Trans. Studies Coll. of Physicians, Philadelphia	*Transactions and Studies of the College of Physicians of Philadelphia*
Trans. Coll. of Physicians, Philadelphia	*Transactions of the College of Physicians of Philadelphia*
Tr. N.Y. Acad. Sci.	*Transactions of the New York Academy of Science*

Univ. Calif. Publications in Am. Archaeology and Ethnology   University of California Publications in American Archaeology and Ethnology

Yale J. Biol. and Med.   Yale Journal of Biology and Medicine

Disease and Its Control

1
THE BIRTH AND DEATH OF DISEASES

"When young men, not yet arrived at their full growth, are forcibly impressed into the military service, and thereby at once lose all hope of returning safe and sound to their beloved homes and country, they become sad, silent, listless, solitary, musing, and full of sighs and moans, and finally quite regardless of, and indifferent to, all the cares and duties of life. From this state of mental disorder nothing can rouse them – neither argument, nor promises, nor the dread of punishment; and the body gradually pines and wastes away. . . . This is the disease nostalgia."

So wrote Leopold Auenbrugger, the eighteenth-century physician who discovered the value of tapping on the chest, or percussion, in detecting diseases of the lungs and heart. Nor, in his view, were the ravages of nostalgia limited to mental alterations. "I have examined the bodies of many youths who have fallen victim to it," Auenbrugger continued, "and have uniformly found the lungs firmly united to the pleura, and the lobes . . . callous, indurated, and more or less purulent."[1]

We now believe that the pathological lungs he encountered

An earlier version of this chapter appeared as Robert P. Hudson, "How Diseases Birth and Die," *Transactions and Studies of the College of Physicians of Philadelphia* 45: 18–27, 1977.

were largely due to tuberculosis, but the mental symptoms Auenbrugger recounted remain common among military draftees. Yet the syndrome would not currently be labeled a disease, and its sufferer would receive none of the special benefits society confers on the ill.

Earlier medical texts abound with diagnostic terms which would be unrecognizable to a medical practitioner today. There was lardaceous liver, gleet, chlorosis, febricula, status thymicus — all terms that conveyed discrete meaning to physicians who used them, but which have since dropped from medical parlance. What were they? What happened to them? How were they born, and why did they die?

Examining the birth and death of diseases can be intrinsically intriguing to medical historians and philosophers, a sort of scholarly whodunit. It can also have direct implications for health professionals and those who pay the costs of health care. This is because many of the processes that operated in the birth and death of older diseases are still in force today. The concept of disease is a dynamic, human creation which is changing now just as it always has. Because our conception of a disease dictates our response to that disease, it becomes incumbent on professionals to understand their personal role as accoucheurs and undertakers, unwitting or not, in the birth and death of conditions labeled as disease. In 1967 the head of the National Institute of Mental Health officially pronounced suicide a disease. The assertion had far-reaching effects. Centers to prevent suicide sprang up, some with the assistance of taxpayers' money. A medical journal, *The Bulletin of Suicidology*, was founded. Conferences were held at which learned men pondered the causes, treatment, and prevention of the new disease. It is reasonable to inquire what brought all of this about. The phenomenon of self-destruction had not changed. It was not as though a virus had mutated into a new and more deadly form of influenza. Yet what had been a sin in the eighteenth century and a crime in the nineteenth was now a disease in the twentieth.

A backward look can illuminate a number of the mechanisms underlying the natality and mortality of diseases. It is possible that identifying these mechanisms can contribute to a better understanding of the evolution of disease as it proceeds around us. It might even assist in social planning, at least to the extent that health professionals and others would pause to consider the consequences of applying the disease label to behavioral deviance and other such social phenomena.

Pondering the birth and death of diseases is by no means a new occupation of the human mind. In ancient Rome, Pliny was certain that he could identify several new diseases, and Plutarch believed that hydrophobia was novel to his time. In the early sixteenth century, almost all physicians were convinced that syphilis had appeared during their lifetime. The great English physician of the seventeenth century, Thomas Sydenham, averred that the influenza of 1688 was a new illness, and in that same century a number of physicians concluded that rickets was absolutely a new disease.

In more recent times a number of students have examined the demise of individual diseases. From these accounts and others it is possible to identify a number of social and natural forces that have caused diseases to come and go.

Environmental Diseases

Because they are obvious to everyone, and because their mechanisms of birth and death are relatively straightforward, the first group to be considered is that of environmental diseases. In this instance, one need not resort to history: a number of environmental diseases have come into existence in our lifetime. Indeed, scarcely a month goes by without a new birth announcement, though it is more difficult to identify environmental diseases that have had a certain demise. Of the hundreds of possible examples we need mention only the insidious nativity between 1953 and 1960 of Minamata Disease, which resulted when a Japanese industrial plant dumped mercury into Minamata Bay. The mystery here was that records supplied by the plant managers indicated they had dumped nothing but inorganic mercury, which is far less toxic to man than the organic form. Scientists then made the terrifying discovery that the tons of inorganic mercury that had been dumped in the world's waters over the years did not always remain inorganic. Rather it could be converted by bacteria into deadly methylmercury, which was then consumed by plankton and passed via fish to human beings.

A subdivision of the environmental category is occupational diseases. These too have a long history, dating, in a definitive sense, to Bernardino Ramazzini, who said in his 1700 publication, *Diseases of Tradesmen,* "We must own that some Arts intail no small mischief upon the respective artisans, and that the same means by which they support Life, and maintain their Families, are oftentimes the cause of grievous Distempers, which hurry them out of the World."[2] In this group are such veteran conditions as berylliosis, from the metal beryllium used in a number of industrial processes, including the manufacture of fluorescent lamps; bagassosis, from inhaling the fibrous material left after sugar has been extracted from sugar cane; byssinosis, from the inhalation of cotton dust; and coal miner's pneumoconiosis, or Black Lung. Newcomers include cancer of the liver in workers handling vinyl chloride, green-tobacco sickness among tobacco harvesters, and respiratory illness in meat wrappers.

The point to be stressed about environmental diseases is an obvious one – they are born when human beings engage in certain activities, and they die when those activities cease or when people take whatever precautions are necessary to separate their physiology from the offending agents. There are, to be sure, a few inescapable disease-producing agents of purely natural origin, such as the solar radiation that contributes to skin cancer, but these are negligible when viewed in the context of environmental disease generally.

Iatrogenic Disease

A second category embraces what are termed iatrogenic diseases. The term iatrogenic literally means physician induced, but for purposes here it will be expanded to include all disease resulting from the application of medical practices, whether by individual physicians, public health programs, or others. The mechanisms of birth and death in iatrogenic diseases are basically identical to those underlying environmental diseases; they are born when patients encounter new diagnostic or therapeutic modalities, and they die when the contact ends. At present the two categories are similar as well in that for each the births far outstrip the deaths.

Iatrogenic conditions can be considered in two categories, real disease and pseudodisease. Real diseases include such conditions as shock from penicillin anaphylaxis and the encephalitis from smallpox vaccination, which was unreported before the present century. Real iatrogenic diseases now constitute a significant portion of the total morbidity in industrialized nations. Their descriptions fill a book of some 500 pages aptly entitled *Diseases of Medical Progress*. They are so widespread and well known that they need no further elaboration here.

Iatrogenic pseudodisease is used to denote the large and fascinating group of diseases that physicians and society over the years defined into and out of existence. Pseudodisease is not to be confused with nondisease, the somewhat whimsical but still thought-provoking term elaborated by Clifton Meador in 1965. Meador informed us that "a nondisease may exist when a specific disease is suspected and when the suspected disease is not found." As evidence he offered fifteen patients he had seen who were slightly obese, middle-aged, with round faces, ruddy complexions, and prominent hair on the upper lip. All were suspected of having Cushing's disease, but laboratory tests ruled out this diagnosis. Meador argued that since these patients did not have Cushing's disease, they had to have Cushing's nondisease, and went on to say:

One might argue that this is ridiculous; the patient happened to have a combination of findings that represented normal variations so that Cushing's disease was only suspected. To the physician unfamiliar with nondisease that is true, but not so for the serious student of health and its classification. Thus, a nondisease exists when a specific entity is suspected but not found. Students of disease only might then argue that all normal persons therefore have non-Cushing's disease. Again this is not valid; not all normal persons are suspected of having Cushing's disease, so how could they have non-Cushing's disease?[3]

Historically the situation is further confused by the finding that Meador's nondisease was indeed previously labelled pseudodisease. In the nineteenth century, for instance, after an iron deficiency anemia was determined as the basis of the disease of young women called chlorosis, physicians continued to encounter patients exhibiting all the signs and symptoms of chlorosis, but not the anemia. For want of a better designation these were diagnosed as pseudochlorosis.

For our purposes pseudodisease will be used to describe a

medical condition which was diagnosed as a disease at one time, but which, for reasons such as improved diagnostic methods, was later abandoned. Historically, pseudodiseases have often been associated with organs whose function is not yet known, organs, so to speak, in search of a disease. The list of deceased pseudodiseases includes such conditions as status thymicolymphaticus, thymic asthma, Pende's syndrome or hyperfunction of the thymus, pineal myopathy, and catarrhal jaundice, which was propounded even by the great clinician Sir William Osler and which was thought to be jaundice due to the swelling and obstruction of the terminal portion of the common bile duct.

There was athlete's heart to account for the large heart and slow pulse now understood as normal in some highly trained athletes; ptomaine poisoning, which was thought to be due to toxic breakdown products of spoiled protein, but which is now held to be bacterial food poisoning; presbycardia or senile heart; and essential gastrorrhagia or stomach bleeding, believed to be a form of vicarious menstruation.

There are diseases whose existence is currently debated, Buerger's disease, for example, which was unquestionably a disease twenty years ago but which is now the subject of considerable dispute. Buerger's disease was first described in 1908 and had an unquestioned existence for fifty years. It occurred in men aged twenty through forty-five, mostly Jewish and almost all tobacco smokers. It caused changes in blood vessels which even the pathologists did not dispute. By 1960, however, it had been concluded that in the decade of the 1950s no patient had been admitted to Boston's Beth Israel Hospital in which a diagnosis of Buerger's disease could be made with certainty. It was recommended that the term be abandoned for diagnostic purposes. Even those who argue that Buerger's disease is a specific entity agree that the incidence is declining rapidly for unknown reasons.

It must not be thought that simply because we now agree a given disease never existed that in fact it did not exist, because of course it did. It existed in its place and time. The distinction between disease and illness as explored in Chapter 11 may help resolve this apparently questionable logic. It is quite fair to say that in terms of today's medical understanding the *disease* catarrhal jaundice never existed, but it does not follow that the *ill-*

ness catarrhal jaundice did not exist, because in practice it did. Patients developed the symptoms of catarrhal jaundice; physicians made the diagnosis, in which other physicians concurred; and the illness was treated the way physicians treated catarrhal jaundice. And these are the elements needed to prove the existence of a given illness, then or now.

Nor must it be imagined that the results of creating a disease were always inconsequential. Around the turn of the twentieth century a prominent pseudodisease was visceroptosis. In this condition, one or more of the viscera, usually the stomach, colon, liver, or kidney, was held to produce symptoms because it had moved down from its proper anatomic location, hence the term visceroptosis. Bernard Shaw parodied the surgical approach to visceroptosis in the *Doctor's Dilemma,* wherein he had surgeons getting rich by removing a mysterious nuciform sac which anatomists, for some reason, were unable to find, though it was easily visible to the trained surgical eye. In 1915 health columnist Logan Clendening admonished the famous British advocate of the surgical correction of visceroptosis, Sir Arbuthnot Lane, as follows: "The modern membranic surgeon goes to his Donnybrook fair every day: 'If you see anything inside the abdomen, do something. If it is tight make it loose, if it is loose, make it tight, untie the organs, let them float, or else on Mondays and Wednesdays and Fridays let us sew them all up to the abdominal parietes.' " Sir Arbuthnot had noted, "An incapacity to perform any mental exercise was a common feature of intestinal stasis," leading Clendening to muse somewhat irreverently, "Has he had his own colon removed may we ask?"[4]

Cultural Diseases

Another category of diseases that are born and die is cultural in nature. Examples of patterns of living that influence our diseases come easily to mind – cirrhosis from alcohol, lung cancer and emphysema from cigarettes, trichinosis from undercooked pork and beef, tularemia or rabbit fever, and hookworm from going barefoot, to mention a few. Perhaps there is no more dramatic and discrete example of a cultural disease than kuru, the deadly nervous system disease found in the Fore people of eastern New Guinea. Kuru is characterized by a staggering gait and the shiver-

ing tremor which gives the disease its name. Usually it pro-
gresses to a total motor incapacity and death within three to nine
months. For years scientists puzzled over the strange malady and
particularly its rarity in adult males. It is now believed that the
disease is caused by a slow-acting virus which is transmitted by
the ritualistic cannibalism which the Fore practice as a sign of
mourning and respect for dead kinsmen. Adult males are infrequently involved because they rarely ingest central nervous tissue. Cannibalization has ended over the past fifteen years, and
the disease has now disappeared among children and adoles-
cents. Presumably the American death rates for lung cancer and
cirrhosis of the liver would diminish from a similar cultural shift
away from the use of tobacco and alcohol.

Cultural pseudodiseases exist as well, a particularly fine historical example being masturbatory insanity. In the eighteenth
century, largely due to the writings of a Swiss physician by the
name of Tissot, masturbation was linked causally to a host of
mental disorders. From this jumbled conglomerate, medical people gradually came to believe that masturbation produced a
specific form of insanity. The heavy hand of religion in medical
beliefs is obvious in this chapter of the story, although physicians were undoubtedly influenced by observing what they took
to be excessive masturbation among asylum inmates. In any
event few physicians of the late nineteenth century doubted the
existence of masturbatory insanity. The "masturbatory personality" was clearly spelled out in Tuke's *Dictionary of Psychological
Medicine.*

The face becomes pale and pasty, and the eye lustreless. The man loses
all spontaneity and cheerfulness, all manliness and self-reliance. He cannot look you in the face because he is haunted by the consciousness of a
dirty secret which he must always conceal. . . . He shuns society, has no
intimate friends, does not dare to marry. . . . [Later he] becomes a liar, a
coward and a sneak . . . [and finally] he sinks into melancholic demen-
tia, relieved only by occasional excitement due to a temporary revival of
his jaded passions.[5]

Perhaps following the medical dictum that dire diseases demand dire remedies, attempts at curing masturbatory insanity
included such heroics as cantharides (oral administration of
dried beetles, which, paradoxically, was also used as an aphro-

disiac), clitoridectomy, castration, and placing a silver ring through the foreskin.

Again, merely because we no longer recognize masturbatory insanity, we may not say that the condition never existed. On the contrary, its certain existence in the nineteenth century is simply a reaffirmation of the fact that disease has no absolute reality, that only illness exists. And again the practices resulting from a particular conception of disease were not innocuous. The precise number of persons, mostly young, who were institutionalized for practicing the "solitary vice" can never be known. We suspect the figure was not inconsiderable. In 1879 a physician reported that nearly 9 percent of the inmates of a large number of insane asylums in the United States carried a diagnosis of masturbatory insanity.

Cultural pseudodiseases can serve the further purpose of illustrating that physicians, in their conception of disease, are often no more immune to their cultural milieu than lay persons. The moral vehemence underlying the medical conception of masturbatory insanity is exemplified in the words of Dr. Henry Maudsley, an English authority on mental disease, who wrote, "Once the habit is formed and the mind has positively suffered from it . . . there would be almost as much hope of the Ethiopian changing his skin, or the leopard its spots, as of his abandoning the vice. . . . the sooner he sinks to his degraded rest the better for himself, and the better for the world which is well rid of him."[6]

Do Diseases Die Naturally?

All the diseases so far considered have related to human activity, either directly or indirectly. They have resulted from cultural practices, occupations, or the activities of physicians, or from a social and medical consensus of sorts that simply defined a disease into existence and out again. It remains to ask, do diseases die *naturally*, by which is meant, totally outside human activities? In truth the question is difficult to phrase in meaningful terms, because it is ultimately impossible to be certain that human activity did not influence the birth or death of a given disease in ways that were not perceived at the time and cannot be reconstructed historically. The terrible sweeps of bubonic plague during and after the fourteenth century would appear to have been a new invasion of foreign bacteria into a susceptible population, and otherwise unrelated to human activity. As we shall see in a later section, however, the epidemics depended, among other factors, on housing practices and crowded conditions that were hospitable to *Rattus rattus,* the flea-bearing house rat, among which an epizootic is necessary to sustain a large outbreak of the plague.

A more modern, though still tenuous, example is the dramatic absolute decline of carcinoma of the stomach in the United States. Forty years ago this tumor was the leading cause of cancer mortality in males in this country – today it is the fifth leading cause among men and eighth in women. There is some evidence that this decline may stem from chemical antioxidant preservatives, notably BHT and BHA, added to breakfast cereals. If this relationship is proved, it will demonstrate that human beings by their actions can unwittingly alter their disease patterns in ways that contemporaries would have attributed to purely natural changes.

So it may not be tenable to speak of historical diseases that were born and died completely apart from the actions of human beings who had the disease. Still the historical picture is far from clear. We have no good evidence of epidemic poliomyelitis before 1840, and no reliable evidence of encephalitis before the eighteenth century. It can be argued that these diseases have always been with us, but without the constellation of conditions necessary to produce an epidemic. Still their symptoms are so distinctive – the permanent wasting paralysis of polio and the prolonged coma in encephalitis – that it is risky to argue that the diseases existed even endemically and were not recognized by such early astute clinicians as Sydenham, Corvisart, and Laennec. But once again cultural and social factors cannot be entirely ruled out. Poliomyelitis in earlier times could have been ubiquitous but limited to the very young, who may have contracted mild cases that conferred permanent immunity. In later times with the improved sanitation that accompanied increasing affluence, the young might have had no early contact with the virus, and thus were susceptible to the paralytic form as young adults. Something akin to this is used to explain the fact that persons living in areas of poor sanitation develop protective antibodies against poliomyelitis at an early age, whereas those in regions of effective sanitary measures do not reach their peak of immunity until age fifteen or older. Lacking the technology to identify viruses and immunity, earlier physicians would have missed the mild childhood cases, and in absence of the severe, paralytic form in young adults, might easily have missed altogether the existence of poliomyelitis.

A consideration of the question of a natural life cycle for diseases leads one sooner or later to the sweating sickness or English Sweate of the fifteenth and sixteenth centuries. While no comprehensive historical treatment of this condition is possible here, the Sweate is useful for at least two reasons. First, it came and went in five great epidemics within a mere sixty-six years, and second, its symptoms were so distinctive that contemporary observers were confident they could diagnose it accurately and date precisely each of its fatal appearances. Although there are disputes about the date of the second and third epidemics, all observers, then and now, agree that the sweating sickness struck England first in 1485 and departed forever after the epidemic that began in 1551. If this is true, then clearly the sweating sickness represents a category of diseases that began and ended apparently outside any human intervention. But is it true?

There were a number of features that combined to make the English Sweate quite unlike any then known epidemic disease. Outstanding among these was its tremendous lethality and remarkably short duration. We do not have accurate mortality figures for this period, but there is no question but what the sweating sickness was deadly. Holinshed, the English chronicler, who lived through one or more of the epidemics, said that scarcely one of every hundred stricken managed to survive. This is probably exaggerated; recent demographic studies suggest that the Sweate produced greater popular terror than similar mortality from bubonic plague. Still its effects were far from negligible. Major feast days were cancelled, Oxford University closed down, and the coronation of Henry VII was postponed. Not even love could overcome the pervasive panic that followed the Sweate. Henry VIII, who was pursuing Anne Boleyn during the 1528 epidemic, had his ardor chilled precipitately when he learned that Anne's chambermaid was stricken with the Sweate. Henry decamped immediately on the first of several flights to avoid the epidemic.

As for its other striking clinical feature, many commentators agreed that the Sweate lasted only twenty-four hours. The outstanding symptoms and signs agreed to by most observers were the sudden onset of a shaking chill, high fever, soaking foul-smelling sweats that might demand twenty to thirty bed changes a night, terrible weakness, headache, palpitation, chest and upper abdominal pain, and finally brain involvement with delirium, coma, and death. All of this at times in twenty-four hours or less.

There were a number of other distinctive features that must be reconciled before we can hope to pin a modern name on the sweating sickness. The disease struck the young and robust more than infants and the aged, groups that we would expect to see die in large numbers had the disease been a particularly virulent form of influenza, as some have postulated. Further, in only one of the five epidemics was the mortality great among the poor. In the other four sweeps the disease was noted as far worse among the wealthy and influential. Third, it came back in waves weeks after the initial spread, suggesting that an attack conferred no immunity, not even a temporary variety. This same phenomenon was frequently described in influenza epidemics before we learned that the apparent recurrences actually were pneumonia secondary to the influenza itself.

Finally we come to the biggest obstacle of all. For two important reasons the pattern of spread was more that of an insect vector disease than one of interpersonal contagion. First, the epidemics usually broke out with the arrival of warm weather and ended in fall or early winter. Second, the pattern followed that of yellow fever or typhus, insect vector diseases, not that of smallpox or influenza, which spread directly from one person to another. That is to say, only one individual in a home might contract the sweating sickness, or it might strike only one home in a block. This is a particularly vexing observation for those who later pointed to the many similarities between sweating sickness and a virulent form of influenza.

The virulence of the sweating sickness simply does not square with any known infectious disease. Among infectious diseases today, only meningitis and poliomyelitis kill with such rapidity and then only rarely. On the basis of this alone we are tempted to conclude that the sweating sickness was a new disease in a susceptible population. The heavy mortality that can result when a people first encounter a contagious disease is a phenomenon well known in the history of disease. It was seen, for example, only a decade after the initial epidemic of sweating sickness when syphilis either first appeared in Europe or assumed a much greater virulency than before. That disease, too, carried an early mortality quite unlike the syphilis we know today. This feature would square with the generally accepted view that sweating sickness came to England with the 2,000 mercenaries Henry brought with him from France and led to victory at the battle of Bosworth Field. But it leaves unanswered the question of how France for many years could harbor an endemic disease to which Englishmen were terribly susceptible, given the large social, commercial, and military intercourse between the two nations over the years.

The disease most often advanced as a possible modern equivalent to the English Sweate is influenza, and it is an attractive possibility. Against this thesis is the absence of prominent catarrhal symptoms, the sporadic skip-about mode of spread already mentioned, and the supposed limitation, except in 1528–1529, to England, a phenomenon quite alien to influenza pandemics of modern times.

A second possible culprit is the spirochetal disease known as relapsing fever, which is transmitted to man by ticks and lice. Only the louse form is capable of producing epidemics. Man gets the disease probably not from the bite, but from crushing the louse on the skin, a perfectly understandable human reaction to the parasite. In 1916 Arpad Gerster championed the position that relapsing fever and the English Sweate were identical. He has not been supported in his contention, which is moderately strange because nothing we have learned about relapsing fever since 1916 has materially weakened his case.

The clinical course of relapsing fever and that of the sweating sickness match reasonably well. Relapsing fever has an insect vector as appeared to be the case with the Sweate. The principal difference is the rapid high mortality of the Sweate, but this, as we have seen, differentiates the Sweate from all known contagious diseases. If the English Sweate was relapsing fever in a highly susceptible population, it calls syphilis immediately to mind. With syphilis we have another spirochetal disease erupting in epidemic form for the first time in Europe, only ten years after the first outbreak of sweating sickness. Whether there is any cross-immunity between the spirochetes of syphilis and relapsing fever is uncertain, though it is known that about 20 percent of victims of relapsing fever do develop a positive serological test for syphilis. This could be an important clue. It might, for example, figure into a population immunity that could help explain the final riddle of the English Sweate – What happened to it after the epidemic of 1551?

Assigning an unequivocal modern diagnostic term to the sweating sickness remains impossible. Contemporary medical men simply were not the meticulous clinical observers physicians would later become. Even their descriptive words have subtle nuances that elude us five hundred years later. Nor of course did they have even the most rudimentary resort to laboratory confirmation. In past historical writings, reference to the English Sweate is almost always preceded by the adjective mysterious. And so it must remain, at least for now.

With the Sweate, then, we confront the possibility, at least, that diseases have their own life cycles. Given this, it would follow that the cycle could be interrupted at any time by a number of mechanisms. The microorganism could mutate into a nonpathogen or to a level of lowered virulence that would produce a symbiotic relationship with its human host. Natural selection could produce a human host with increased immunity, thus achieving symbiosis from another direction. Finally, of course, the germ of sweating sickness, if it was a germ, could indeed have died out. Such an end has befallen many species of animals throughout the course of time. If the massive dinosaur could become extinct, there is no reason the same may not have happened to any number of microscopic species. At the moment, as noted, we can only suspend judgment.

Still, an overweening pessimism is not called for. History, it has been said, purifies itself like running water, a fact our temporal arrogance at times leads us to forget. One striking feature of the sweating sickness that has not been dwelled on before is the remarkable periodicity of the five known epidemics. As mentioned earlier there are variations of one year involving the second and third outbreaks, depending on whose dates are accepted. If Zinsser's dates are employed, that is, 1485, 1507, 1518, 1529, and 1551, the epidemics were separated by intervals of 22, 11, 11, and 22 years, which is to say by 11 years or a multiple thereof. One need not revert to astrology to wonder about possible cosmic influences in an otherwise remarkable coincidence. The study of cosmic and meteorologic influences on human disease is only in its infancy, but it is being pursued by serious scientists. There is evidence, for instance, that human fertility is more related to meteorologic conditions than cultural factors. To flirt with science fiction, a liaison scientists have found vastly rewarding at times, one might point out that sunspots also demonstrate eleven-year cycles, the peaks of which greatly increase the amount of cosmic radiation reaching the Earth's atmosphere. In this regard it might be recalled that the most serious recent pandemics of influenza occurred in 1946, 1957, and 1968, also intervals of eleven years. How sunspots might alter meteorologic factors, or human immunity, or microbial mutations in ways that contribute to periodicity in eruptions of epidemic diseases must be left to further running of the historical river. It is, however, brought up in complete seriousness. The fact that we get further away in time from the epidemics of sweating sickness is no reason in itself to despair of a final solution. Advances in our understanding of diseases in general may one day give us far more secure grounds on which to decide whether the sweating sickness is an example of a disease that died, and if so, whether the death was permanent or whether diseases indulge in something akin to reincarnation.

Legionnaires' Disease

Before leaving the question of how diseases are born and die, the outbreak of Legionnaires' disease in Philadelphia in 1976 deserves passing attention. This small epidemic has had the paradoxical effect of diminishing our confidence in our ability to identify the causes of past epidemics, and at the same time of comforting us in our ignorance. If a peerless Center for Disease Control could be totally baffled for five months by an apparently new disease in 1976, the failures of physicians to identify the causes of epidemics in the prebacteriologic era become eminently understandable.

After the organism responsible for Legionnaires' disease was identified, it turned out that we were not dealing with a new disease at all. Epidemiologic and immunologic evidence soon made it highly likely that the same bacterium had been responsible for outbreaks of pneumonia in the District of Columbia in 1965; in Pontiac, Michigan, in 1968; and in Philadelphia in 1974. Thus Legionnaires' disease was not an example of the birth of a new disease, but merely the identification of a form of pneumonia that had been improperly classified in the past.

The public has great faith in the powers of medical science, and here again Legionnaires' disease is instructive. The first cases began appearing in July and August of 1976. Yet scientists at the Center for Disease Control, working under heavy public pressure, could not announce a tentative solution of the mystery until January 18, 1977. In the wake of the furor aroused by the Legionnaires' outbreak, it turned out that a dozen mini-epidemics were investigated in the ten years after 1966 in which no cause was ever discovered. The twelve outbreaks involved more than 7,800 persons in various parts of the country and at sea. They received none of the publicity accorded the Legionnaires' episode because only two involved deaths, one killing five persons, the other sixteen.

Not only should such unsolved epidemics render us more forgiving of our medical ancestors and their attempts at sorting out and dealing with diseases, but they should make us more wary of the names they used and of our ability to solve such puzzles with nothing more than the rational process, armed with the medical knowledge that has accumulated since Henry VII and his troops apparently first brought the Sweate to England in 1485.

Comfort derives from our initial failure in putting together the many puzzling aspects of the Legionnaires' event, because it demonstrates just how complex the appearance of an apparently new disease can be. Two years after the bacterial culprit was identified, the way by which Legionnaires' disease spread remained unsolved. Infectious disease experts and historians of diseases need not be humiliated by the circumstances surrounding Legionnaires' disease, but it is altogether proper that they be humbled.

Notes

1. Camac, C.N.B. *Classics of Medicine and Surgery*. New York: Dover Publications, 1959, p. 132.
2. Ramazzini, B. *Diseases of Tradesmen*. H. Goodman, ed. New York: Medical Lay Press, 1933, p. 22.
3. Meador, C. K. "The Art and Science of Nondisease," *New Eng J. Med.* 272:92-95, 1965.
4. Clendening, L. "A Review of the Subject of Chronic Intestinal Stasis," *Interstate Med. J.* 22:4, 9, 1915.
5. Tuke, H. *A Dictionary of Psychological Medicine*. London: J. & A. Churchill, 1892, p. 784.
6. Maudsley, H. "Illustrations of a Variety of Insanity," *J. Mental Sci.*, July 1868, pp. 153-161. In Skultans, V. *Madness and Morals: Ideas on Insanity in the Nineteenth Century*. London: Routledge & Kegan Paul, 1975, p. 94.

Bibliographic Commentary

Over the years a number of studies have appeared dealing with the appearance and disappearance of diseases. Among these are D. Riesman, "Deceased Diseases," *Ann. Med. Hist.* 8:160-167, 1936; B. Straus, "Defunct and Dying Diseases," *Bull. N.Y. Acad. Med.* 46:686-706, 1970; and R. P. Hudson, "How Diseases Birth and Die," *Tr. and Studies, Coll. of Physicians of Phila.* 45:18-27, 1977.

Somewhat more specialized treatments that still have general implications are H. Rolleston, "Changes in the Character of Diseases," *Brit. Med. J.* 1:499-500, 1933; L. G. Stevenson, " 'New Diseases' in the Seventeenth Century," *Bull. Hist. Med.* 39:1-21, 1965; R. P. Hudson, "The Biography of Disease: Lessons from Chlorosis," *Bull. Hist. Med.* 51:448-463, 1977; and S. Jarcho, "Some Lost, Obsolete, or Discontinued Diseases: Serous Apoplexy, Incubus, and Retrocedent Ailments," *Tr. and Studies, Coll. of Physicians of Phila.* 2:241-266, 1980.

The basic problem of retrospective diagnosis was discussed by C. J. Hackett in E. Clarke, ed., *Modern Methods in the History of Medicine*, London: The Athalone Press, 1971. Tuberculosis and nostalgia are discussed in J. Starobinski, "Le Nostalgie: Théories Médicales et Expression Littéraire," *Studies on Voltaire and the Eighteenth Century* 27:1505-1518, 1963. The only exhaustive compilation of iatrogenic illness is R. H. Moser's *Diseases of Medical Progress*, Springfield, Ill.: Charles C. Thomas, 1969.

The story of kuru can be found in D. C. Gajdusek, "Unconventional Viruses and the Origin and Disappearance of Kuru," *Science* 197:943-960, 1977; and J. Farquhar and D. C. Gajdusek, eds., *Kuru: Early Letters and Field-Notes from the Collection of D. Carleton Gajdusek.* New York: Raven Press, 1981.

The seminal article on masturbatory insanity was E. H. Hare, "Masturbatory Insanity: The History of an Idea," *J. Mental Sci.* 108:1-25, 1962. An excellent account from a disease orientation is H. T. Engelhardt, Jr., "The Disease of Masturbation: Values and the Concept of Disease," *Bull. Hist. Med.* 48:234-248, 1974.

There is an extensive literature on the English Sweate. An English translation of John Caius's sixteenth-century description of the sweating sickness is in R. H. Major, *Classic Descriptions of Disease,* Springfield, Ill.: Charles C. Thomas, 1932. The older literature includes J.F.C. Hecker, *The Epidemics of the Middle Ages,* London: The Sydenham Society, 1846; A. G. Gerster, "What Was the English Sweating Sickness or Sudor Anglicus of the Fifteenth and Sixteenth Centuries?" *Johns Hopkins Hosp. Bull.* 27:332-337, 1916; H. Zinsser, *Rats, Lice and History,* Boston: Little, Brown & Company, 1935; and C. Creighton, *A History of Epidemics in Britain,* London: Frank Cass & Co., 1965.

A recent demographic study of the Sweate is R. S. Gottfried, "Population, Plague, and the Sweating Sickness: Demographic Movements in Late Fifteenth-Century England," *J. Brit. Studies* 17:12-37, 1977. For evidence of the persistent difficulty in assigning a modern diagnostic term to the Sweate, see A. Patrick, "A Consideration of the Nature of the English Sweating Sickness," *Med. Hist.* 9:272-279, 1965; and a refutation by R. S. Roberts in the same volume, pp. 385-389.

An entire issue of *Ann. Int. Med.* was devoted to the story of Legionnaires' disease (90:492-714, 1979).

2
DISEASE AND HISTORY

Individual Illness

"A difference," someone once said, "to be a difference, must make a difference." In later pages we will find that over the centuries profound differences have characterized Western views of disease and its management. Before considering that story it should be asked if such differences have made a difference or, put another way, to what extent has disease influenced the course of history? The question can be examined from the standpoint of episodes of illness in individuals and by considering mass, or epidemic, disease.

The question of whether individual illness has altered the course of history has as a corollary the ancient question of men shaping events versus events shaping men. We might begin by asking the reader to think back to a recent indisposition. It need not have been serious—a bout of flu, a migraine headache, menstrual cramps, or even a rollicking good hangover will do. Recall what the ailment did to your intellectual processes and your will for action. Unless you are an exceptional stoic, you will probably agree that human beings do not function ideally in the face of pain, or nausea, or chills and fever, or severe depression, or any of the "thousand natural shocks that flesh is heir to." If we agree that even minor discomforts can disrupt normal function, it follows that disease must have influenced some of the decisions and actions of those who have made history. Yet when the record is consulted, not much is found on the subject. Historians generally have downplayed the role personal disease may have played in the story of humankind.

There are reasons that help explain the paucity of reference to disease in the writings of political and economic historians. Prior to the nineteenth century diagnosis was a confused and uncertain business. The diseases that written records connect with important persons in earlier times were not always accurately diagnosed. Certain more dramatic and distinctive conditions, such as epilepsy, could be identified with confidence, but even here we now know what writers in previous centuries could not know, that the symptoms of epilepsy can be caused by a variety of underlying conditions, ranging from minor scarring of the brain to malignant tumors.

Even when a prominent person can be linked to a given disease, often there is no way to assess the effect of the disease on the person's actions. Syphilis, because of its venereal origin and characteristic first stage ulcer, is a disease which could be identified with reasonable accuracy in previous centuries. The list of persons who reportedly contracted syphilis reads like a sort of venereal *Who's Who*, although the ultimate uncertainty of the diagnosis must be reiterated. Among rulers there was Henry III and Charles VIII of France, Christian VII of Denmark, Frederick the Great, Ivan the Terrible, and Peter the Great. Churchmen include Pope Alexander VI and Leo X. In the creative world are listed Erasmus, Dürer, Cellini, Gauguin, Van Gogh, de Maupassant, Marlowe, Boswell, Wilde, Heine, Schumann, Paganini, Beethoven, and Schopenhauer. For these individuals we lack an accurate day-to-day clinical account of their symptoms and thus have no way of assessing the role disease may have played in their lives or how it may have helped determine the nature of their contributions.

But these reasons alone seem not to explain fully the historical neglect of disease in individuals. An important piece of the explanation appears to lie in the neglect of disease by historians themselves. In this regard, the case of Woodrow Wilson can be instructive. Wilson was elected twenty-eighth president of the

United States in 1912. As early as 1896, while on the faculty of Princeton University, he had exhibited evidence of disease in the arteries supplying blood to his brain. In May of that year he suffered an episode of weakness and pain in his right arm and numbness of his fingers on that side. It was not until March of 1897 that he could again write smoothly with his right hand.

But a greater catastrophe awaited. On May 28, 1906, Wilson, now president of Princeton, awoke blind in his left eye. A contemporary ophthalmologist diagnosed a ruptured retinal blood vessel, but a later interpretation suggests a more serious generalized disease of the arteries. The combination of right-sided hemiparesis (partial paralysis of one side) and left-sided blindness was probably due to a blocking of the left internal carotid artery, the main supplier of blood to that side of the brain. Wilson never recovered full vision in his left eye, and another attack of right-sided numbness followed in 1908. From 1906 on, intimates noted that Wilson was more irritable, impulsive, aggressive, and intolerant of criticism, behavioral changes characteristic of developing disease in the cerebral arteries.

In early April, 1919, while in Paris leading the peace talks, Wilson experienced another illness, which some believe represented further cerebral vascular disease, although the evidence here is too scanty to allow a comfortable judgment.

The word apoplexy, or stroke, means to strike away, at times into insensibility. Wilson's blow came in September, 1919. The president desperately wanted American approval of the Treaty of Versailles and participation in the League of Nations. His problem lay in the Senate, where ratification had to occur, and the Upper House had narrowly gone to the opposing Republicans in the election of 1918. In an attempt to husband popular support for ratification, Wilson undertook a series of speeches that spanned the country and brought him back to Pueblo, Colorado, where apoplexy struck. There, on September 25, he required help getting on the speaking platform; his voice was weak and mumbling; and he appeared to have trouble tracking his thoughts. One noted physician, listening to Wilson on the radio, diagnosed a stroke on the spot. The next morning his secretary, Joseph Tumulty, found Wilson sitting in a chair, his entire left side paralyzed.

The sad entourage returned to Washington, hiding all information on the nature and extent of Wilson's disability. He began improving, but on October 2, in the presence of his wife, he suffered a more profound and this time permanent stroke. His later years were generally marked by obscurity. Physically unable to run for a third term, he retired to a quiet life in Washington, exercised an admirable restraint regarding political comment, and died in his sleep on February 3, 1924.

At the Paris peace conference it was Wilson's persuasive influence that had brought the contending nations close enough together to permit compromise, though they were not all happy over the outcome. Yet, for Wilson's hopes for his own nation, his efforts came to naught. The United States never joined the Laegue of Nations, in part because Wilson was stricken at an absolutely critical juncture.

But the story is not all that simple. Wilson's personality was in many ways his greatest obstacle. His hated adversary, Senator Henry Cabot Lodge, came to personify the idea of compromise, and Wilson became implacable. In the end he could not even bring himself to release his Senate supporters to follow their own consciences, a move which likely would have taken the United States into the League of Nations. What remains unanswered in all this is the degree to which Wilson's inflexibility and other counterproductive aspects of his personality may have been the result of the disease of his arteries rather than of his genes and life experiences. What also must remain unresolved is the question of what would have transpired had Wilson's second stroke been fatal rather than disabling. One commentator summarized:

Had Wilson died, the Democrats would probably have agreed to reservations; the United States might then have been a member of the League; Wilson, a martyr – his peroration at Pueblo a fitting final testament. As it was, the imprisoned shadow of a once noble man cast across his work and reputation a dreadful pall. . . . Wilson at his healthy best brought the treaty to the shoals. Wilson at his crippled worst steered it to disaster. This was sad for him, his country, and the world.[1]

A finely wrought estimate, but not all historians would agree that Woodrow Wilson was at either his healthiest or his best when he "brought the treaty to the shoals." At that point he had been suffering progressive cerebral vascular disease for at least two decades.

Among American presidents, Wilson's story is by no means exceptional. Of the thirteen presidents since Taft, seven suffered significant disease while in office. Harding had arteriosclerotic heart disease with recurrent bouts of the characteristic chest pain, angina pectoris. As the only one of the seven ailing presidents to die in office, he was probably carried off by a myocardial infarction, which follows the closing down of the blood supply to a portion of the heart muscle. Coolidge, never physically strong, had multiple allergic symptoms, including those of bronchial asthma. These probably contributed to his renowned short working day, as well as his decision not to stand for reelection in 1928. Franklin Roosevelt suffered severe hypertensive heart disease and reportedly died of a cerebral hemorrhage. Eisenhower had a heart attack in 1955 and underwent surgery for regional ileitis in June 1956. Kennedy incurred a severe back reinjury in World War II and suffered from Addison's disease of unknown severity. Before becoming President, Lyndon Johnson had a severe myocardial infarction in 1955, and at his autopsy in 1973, two of the three main coronary arteries were found to be completely occluded. In 1965 he had an acute gall bladder attack requiring surgical removal of that organ, an event which a close aide believed contributed to the "leadership malaise" some thought they detected in Johnson at the time.

Although the degree to which disease affects function in a given leader is impossible to fix with precision, except in such dire circumstances as Wilson's stroke, to deny disease any role at all in determining the events of history flies in the face of medical understanding, to say nothing of ordinary sense.

Epidemic Disease and History

It is difficult for the mind of a modern Westerner to grasp the profound social and psychological impact occasioned by epidemic disease in the past. Due to public health measures and improved nutrition we now enjoy lives largely free of outbreaks of poliomyelitis, measles, diphtheria, yellow fever, bubonic plague, malaria, tuberculosis, leprosy, cholera, typhoid, typhus, and smallpox, diseases which through the centuries carried off millions of persons. Today many citizens of industrialized nations reach middle age or even old age without having suffered a single serious episode of illness. It was not always so. In truth it was not so until the present century. What follows will examine the effect epidemic disease has had upon exploration and settlement, military campaigns, and upon the entire fabric of society as medieval peoples confronted bubonic plague and the other Horsemen of the Apocalypse.

Exploration and Settlement

The manner whereby disease influenced routes of exploration can be seen in the story of scurvy and the settlement of California. Scurvy results from the body's inability to synthesize vitamin C, an inborn error of metabolism shared by all human beings. The deficiency prevents cartilage from turning to bone, loosens teeth, produces painful bleeding, particularly into joints, and leads to death by mechanisms that are poorly understood.

Surprisingly, the fact that citrus fruits could cure scurvy was widely known in the sixteenth and seventeenth centuries, but it was not until after the work of British naval surgeon James Lind in the eighteenth century that citrus products were widely adopted by the maritime world. We will return to Lind in greater detail when we consider the concept of specific therapy. Here it is enough to say that until some two centuries ago, on all long voyages, scurvy was the scourge of the seafaring man. In 1585 Sir Francis Drake set out in quest of Spanish booty with 2,300 men aboard. Within three months some 300 perished, and he lost another 260 before the voyage ended.

Because scurvy made the sea route so treacherously long the Spaniards decided to settle California by land. The mission outposts established in this adventure developed into some of the major urban centers of California today. Indeed it was scurvy that gave early impetus to the citrus industry of California and eventually to the fact that farming there did not go through the forty acres per man that characterized the middle west, but rather depended on large scale operations from the outset.

Even after a sea voyage was completed, the ensuing settlements remained vulnerable to the ravages of scurvy. Colonists in

Quebec, Newfoundland, Virginia, and Hudson's Bay, lacking fresh fruits and vegetables, all suffered heavy casualties from scurvy during early winters there. But the suffering was minor compared to the havoc their infectious diseases wreaked on the natives of North and South America. Unique devastation often follows when an infectious disease is introduced into a population for the first time. The reason is largely a matter of immunity. Not only does a given attack of smallpox usually produce life-long immunity, but persons born into a population in which smallpox is common often inherit a basic immunity which renders them more likely to survive the initial attack. Even diseases which are mild in a regularly exposed population can be lethal in populations which have never been exposed before. In the early seventeenth century smallpox decimated entire tribes of Amerindians. The Massachusetts and Narragansetts dropped from 30,000 and 9,000 respectively to a few hundreds. The 1837 epidemic reduced the Mandans from 1,600 to 31 while the Plains tribes lost some 10,000 members in a disastrous few weeks. The same devastation was recorded during the settlement of California. The smallpox epidemic of 1844 alone reportedly took 100,000 to 300,000 native lives.

Fortunately for the colonists, God was on their side in these matters. The Reverend Cotton Mather, who also practiced medicine, thanked the Divine Hand for landing the Mayflower at a point "wonderfully prepared for their Entertainment by a sweeping Mortality that had lately been among the natives . . . which carried away not a tenth but *Nine Parts of Ten* (yea 'tis said *Nineteen of Twenty*) among them; So that the woods were almost cleared of those pernicious creatures to make room for a better growth."[2] Unless Columbus brought syphilis to Europe from the New World, this early and inadvertent form of bacteriologic warfare was strictly one-sided. In what has been called the Columbian Exchange, no epidemics of similar magnitude were imported from America to Europe.

Disease and War

In his *Devil's Dictionary*, war was defined by Ambrose Bierce as a "by-product of the arts of peace." And so it seems when one

considers the millions of young lives lost in the periodic reshuf-
fling of national boundaries in Europe, or ponders the estimate
that we have known only 268 years of peace in the 3,421 years of
recorded history.

When explaining the outcome of a given battle, generals (and
too often those who write about generals) are wont to emphasize
a brilliant maneuver, a crack regiment, or superior terrain. The
fact is that in many instances battle has been decided by disease,
and not by traditional military activities. Reportedly the first
war in which more soldiers died of martial activities than disease
was the Russo-Japanese conflict of 1904–1905, and this among
the Japanese only. For most of history the larger battles were
fought as sieges, "wolf-strategy" it was called. The enemy was
surrounded, cut off from all assistance, and held in place. Starvation and disease did the rest.

A few statistics will make the point that disease has shaped
many military adventures and, indeed, decided the outcome of
more than one. The Boer War lasted some two and a half years,
during which the British lost an estimated 8,000 troops in battle
and 14,000 from disease. Typhoid fever alone reportedly afflicted 57,684 and killed 8,022. In America's Civil War the first
battle of Vicksburg was almost certainly decided by disease, in
this case principally malaria. A Union victory at Vicksburg could
easily have shortened the war, but after assessing the dismal
health of his men, the Union leader saw the hopelessness of his
situation and postponed any further action until the fever season
ended. So it was that the Mississippi River remained closed for
another year.

Many diseases are commonly associated with war – malaria,
typhoid fever, dysentery, and cholera – diseases easily spread
through contaminated food and water or inadequate waste disposal, or when men are crowded together and susceptible to insects such as mosquitos. But among the microbial scourges
known to attack military combatants, typhus fever deserves special recognition. Typhus has always been the soldier's enemy, in
fact a human nemesis any time large numbers of people are
brought together in unhygienic conditions. Its many names attest to this fact. At different times and in various places, it has
been called war plague, gaol fever, ship fever, lazaret fever (after

the isolation hospitals of the Middle Ages), and even, with grim good reason, hospital fever.

Epidemic typhus is caused by a microorganism named *Rickettsia prowazeki*, a parasite of the human body louse, which it ultimately kills. The louse has an unfortunate proclivity for defecating while it sucks blood from its human host. The feces contain the germ, which is then rubbed into the skin through the feeding punctures by the understandable scratching on the part of the human host. The louse is fastidious where temperature is concerned. When the host's temperature goes up with fever or down with death, the louse departs in search of a more congenial clime, and thus the epidemic spreads.

Within ten to fourteen days of infection, the often fatal scenario begins unfolding – fever, generalized aches and pains, skin rash, delirium, stupor, coma, death. The skin rash is caused by tiny hemorrhages (petechiae), and it is this phenomenon that gives typhus its other popular name, spotted fever.

Many examples of the critical importance of typhus and warfare could be cited, but one will suffice. Three years before Waterloo, Napoleon received a telling lesson on the subject of epidemic disease and warfare. In June of 1812 the Corsican Colossus plunged into Russia with an army of something more than 150,000 men. When he began his retreat from Moscow in October, his contingent of able-bodied men was reduced to 80,000, and on down to an incredible 5,000 by the time he reached Wilno. The Third Army Corps had only twenty men remaining.

The popular notion is that Napoleon was defeated by the bitter Russian winter, and he himself attributed the debacle to "General January." Certain it is that the cold contributed to his defeat, at least near the end of the campaign, but less directly than through its role in spreading typhus. There was no hope of practicing even elemental personal hygiene in a retreat now verging on a rout and in weather that precluded bathing or washing of clothes. On this already dangerous scene came infestation with the body louse and its passenger, the germ of typhus. Although other diseases contributed, typhus was the real nemesis, and a strong argument can be made that Napoleon's grip on Europe was shattered more by this invisible foe than by any other single factor, military or political. On one occasion in conversation with Goethe, Napoleon revealed his belief in the overarching power of men to change history, his conviction that politics are destiny. Politics may be destiny, but so is the lowly body louse.

Microbial devastation in wartime is not limited to those in uniform; civilian populations suffer as well. During Napoleon's retreat, the soldiers served as a reservoir of infection for the surrounding population. As the troops fanned out in search of food, shelter, and medical attention, they infected cities and towns all over central Europe. For the period of Bonaparte's retreat and immediately thereafter, the estimate is that East Prussia alone lost 20,000 persons to typhus. Russian civilians suffered even more terribly in World War I, when typhus killed an estimated 3,000,000 persons. The number of noncombatants dead in Russia during that holocaust from starvation, disease, and other privation exceeded the total killed in battle by all belligerents. To put the matter in perspective it should be recalled that World War I was one of the deadliest ever fought; the number of combatants dead from all causes among the Allies and the Central Powers was placed at 8,538,315. If, as Victor Hugo said, "The success of war is gauged by the amount of damage it does," then World War I has to rank among the more triumphant of mankind's martial adventures.

Bubonic Plague in the Middle Ages

No epoch in Western history has been more scarred by disease than that of Europe from the fourteenth to the sixteenth centuries. The principals in this story were leprosy, plague, and syphilis. Rather than attempt a synthesis of the collective impact of these three diseases, the focus here will be on the one that had the profoundest effect. Bubonic plague is perhaps the best example of how an epidemic disease can influence all aspects of a society, altering economic patterns, cultural practices, medical thought, religious dominance, and even the nature of the arts. Plague also offers an opportunity to examine the question: Could it happen again? Could an epidemic so vast return to an industrialized and scientifically sophisticated Western world in the twentieth century?

It is close to the mark to note that the Middle Ages began and ended with the plague.* The great epidemic that weakened the Roman Empire under Justinian in the sixth century was almost certainly bubonic plague, and after centuries of apparent inactivity, plague returned to Europe in the terrible recurrent waves of the fourteenth century. As we shall see, the degree of historical impact that plague had on medieval society is warmly disputed. No one is rash enough to suggest that plague did nothing to alter life in the Middle Ages, but some scholars now contend that earlier historians tended to exaggerate the effects of the disease on its time. Examining this question will be facilitated by a brief survey of our current understanding of the epidemiology and pathology of the plague.

The reader investigating the history of plague will find the offending germ listed as *Pasteurella pestis* in honor of the great French scientist, Louis Pasteur. That honor has now been removed to Pasteur's student, the true discoverer of the plague bacillus, Alexandre Yersin, hence the current designation, *Yersinia pestis*. The bacterium is normally a parasite of rodents, most importantly for our purpose, *Rattus rattus*, the common black house rat, and invades the human bloodstream only in an incidental fashion. The intermediary that spreads the plague bacillus between rats, or between rats and man, is a rat-flea, the most dangerous being the Asiatic variety, *Xenopsylla cheopis*. The bacterium gains access to the bloodstream through the flea bite, although under certain circumstances the germ travels from person to person directly by way of the respiratory tract. The two important types of plague are the bubonic, in which the portal of entry is the bloodstream, and the pneumonic, in which the germ travels on infectious droplets from coughing or sneezing.

When an infected flea bites a rat, the injected *Y. pestis* multiplies rapidly, producing "blood poisoning" or septicemia. When a second flea feeds on this infected rat, it draws in large numbers

---

*Historically the words *plague* and *pestilence* can be confusing. At times they denote bubonic plague and at other times they are used generically to indicate any epidemic disease. In this book *plague* refers to bubonic plague, and *pestilence* is used in the broader sense.

of bacteria, and in a small proportion of cases, the germ begins multiplying in the flea's stomach. Rather quickly the bacteria completely fill that organ, producing what is termed a blocked flea. Even though its stomach is full, the flea is effectively starving. Driven by hunger, the flea may lose its preference for its usual rodent host and attack any animal at hand, including man. The flea sucks human blood until the distended stomach can stretch no further, at which point it regurgitates and the blood – now mixed with plague bacilli – reenters the human host. As a plague victim dies, whether rat or man, the flea, which prefers a narrow range of temperature, abandons the chilling body in search of a living host. In an infested house, when the rats are all dead or dying, the flea turns then to the next convenient host, the human inhabitants.

A blocked flea can remain alive for up to six weeks, but is probably infective for only some fourteen days during this time. This explains why outbreaks of plague were linked at times to shipments of rags, wool, hides, or other merchandise, a phenomenon noted by contemporaries even though they could not explain their observation. The great European epidemics usually broke out in spring, peaked in summer, diminished in autumn, and effectively disappeared in winter, facts reflecting the key role of the flea, which hibernates in frosty weather.

In modern epidemics, direct human-to-human spread of plague has not been an important element in sustaining a given outbreak. Indeed, a characteristic of these episodes has been the fact that no more than one member of a family contracts the disease. This is because the disease produces such a low level of septicemia in humans that the rat flea does not suck up enough bacteria to establish growth in the flea's stomach. A problem here is that certain medieval observers were absolutely confident that plague spread directly between susceptible persons. Recent demographic works shed at least a ray of light on this apparent contradiction by showing that in one series of fifty-two stricken medieval families, fifty had more than one case per family. From this and other evidence an investigator concluded that certain medieval epidemics of plague were fueled by the human flea rather than the one which favors *Rattus rattus.*[3]

An epidemic in a nonhuman population is termed an epizootic.

In our current understanding an epizootic of plague must have preceded and coincided with every major human outbreak of the disease. The rat portion of our epidemiological equation helps explain why medieval plague struck the poor more than the well-to-do. The poor lived in one-story huts whose thatched roofs were ideal for rat infestation. The wealthy could afford stone or wooden homes with solid roofs, which the domestic rat found far less hospitable.

Of the two important clinical forms of plague, bubonic and pneumonic, bubonic has been the most important. In part this is because an epidemic of the pneumonic form cannot begin or sustain itself in the absence of a coexistent bubonic outbreak. The word bubonic comes from bubo, the name given an infected lymph gland. The location of the enlarged glands depends on the site of bacterial entry; if on the upper leg, for example, the swellings would first appear in the groin. An affected lymph gland can become secondarily infected by pus-producing bacteria, the result being an extremely painful swelling that may then break down and drain outside the skin. Before antibiotics were available, the fatality rate was between 60 and 90 percent, death coming from circulatory collapse.

In the pneumonic form, pneumonia occurs in a person suffering bubonic plague. Thereafter, infection from person to person may occur directly via respiratory droplets. Plague pneumonia is one of the most deadly bacterial infections of man. Untreated cases rarely survive longer than three days, and death within twenty-four hours is not uncommon. It was this form which a number of medieval commentators described so vividly and with such understandable awe. Plague is now treatable with a number of antibiotics. Death in the United States, when it occurs, is usually because the rarity of the disease leads to its omission from the differential diagnosis.

The reason plague made no devastating incursions into Europe between Justinian's era and the fourteenth century probably relates to the matter of animal and human densities. An epizootic cannot exist in rats until a certain minimum population density is exceeded. Similarly, it is not until human beings begin crowding together that the epizootic in rats can become an epidemic in man. The best information has it that plague cannot spread by rat contact where there are fewer than sixty persons per square mile. In fourteenth-century Europe all the necessary conditions were in place. When the plague bacillus entered Sicily in 1347, it found the *ménage à trois* needed to sustain an epidemic – people, rats, and fleas living together as a biologically related family.

One rarely sees mention of bubonic plague without its other designation, the Black Death. Indeed the latter is perhaps more common than the former. Black Death has an attractive dramatic ring, but the phrase is historically and medically misleading. It was not used by those who lived through the plague years, and it does not describe plague victims with any clinical accuracy. In Britain contemporary observers called the plague either "Great Mortality" or "the Great Pestilence," and in Italy the first sweep of 1348 was termed the "universal plague," to distinguish it from earlier epidemics that were not bubonic plague. The phrase Black Death apparently did not appear until the nineteenth century. Medically speaking, Black Death is also a misnomer because plague victims, in life or death, turn no blacker than do sufferers of other microbial diseases. Many dead bodies, whatever the cause, may turn a slate blue or dusky gray, and some fulminant cases of smallpox may even have a charred look, but plague has no particular claim to its popular appellation, the Black Death.

Medieval Explanations

It goes without saying that medieval man knew nothing of the true nature of bubonic plague. The isolation of the responsible germ, the understanding of the rat as host and flea as human vector, the development of a preventive and an effective treatment were all accomplishments of the late nineteenth and twentieth centuries. As socialized people have always done, medieval man had to work his explanation of the origin of the plague into his existing frames of reference. In general, explanations assumed two forms, one religious, the other secular or medical. Because the Church was a far more pervasive and powerful influence than science at the time, it is not surprising to find that the ecclesiastical opinion of plague's etiology held dominion.

The superstitious mind of medieval man may have had no way

to grasp the bionomics of plague spread, but he was certain of the ultimate cause – his own sins. The precise nature of his guilt may at times have seemed vague, but the general burden was everywhere and oppressive. If he ever flagged in this conviction, it was not for long; there was incessant reinforcement from clerics on high. Under such circumstances the plague was readily perceived as nothing more than a particularly devastating manifestation of God's remedial powers.

The medieval medical explanation of the plague's origin is scarcely less alien to twentieth-century thought. To their credit physicians, almost to a man, insisted that the plague was a natural rather than a divine visitation. Further, they required but short acquaintance with the plague to become convinced that it was contagious. They did not think in terms of infection by tiny living organisms, the *contagium animatum* or animalcular theory that would come later. Rather they believed that the disease spread by an altered chemical quality of the atmosphere, an entity that came to be called a miasma and figured prominently in medical thinking well into the nineteenth century. As to the reason for the deadly pollution of the atmosphere, physicians resorted to cosmic influences, but of a natural rather than supernatural ilk. The ultimate cause was deemed to be astrological. The Paris Faculty fixed the fatal conjunction between Mars, Jupiter, and Saturn in the sign of Aquarius, which occurred on March 20, 1345, at one o'clock in the afternoon. This unequivocal pronouncement was thereafter firmly rooted in European medical explanations of the plague. In passing it should be noted that physicians were not thereby forsaking their science; astrology was an integral part of scientific medicine at the time.

Plague Mortality

If one is to argue that bubonic plague had a significant impact on medieval history, the final mortality of the disease assumes obvious importance. The extent and causes of the population decline in England from the early fourteenth century to 1450, for example, have been thoroughly studied, but the entire matter remains one of dispute. The confusion is readily understandable.

Excepting a few cases, accurate mortality figures simply were not compiled for the time in question. In addition, the figures that are available do not distinguish accurately between deaths from plague and other diseases, such as typhus fever. Also basic to the problem is the fact that the Middle Ages demonstrated nothing like our modern infatuation with statistics. On the contrary, the medieval mind was marked by an almost intentional vagueness in the face of large numbers. In England in 1371, for example, the bishops were expelled from the high offices of the church by laymen, who promptly decided to raise £50,000 by a tax on all the parishes in the country. The tax was apportioned on the available information that there were 40,000 parishes in all. As it turned out there were fewer than 9,000, a discrepancy astounding to those who levy taxes nowadays. Another problem is that Roman numeration was retained during most of the Middle Ages even after Arabic numerals were known. Roman numerals do not lend themselves well to large numbers, or for that matter to mathematical manipulation of any kind, as one can discover by trying to multiply LXXXII by CXII or divide MCCLXI by XLII.

The result of all this is that the contemporary estimates of plague mortality were generally overdrawn. A contemporary rhyme indicates the exaggerated nature of estimates at the time:

> In thirteen hundred and forty-eight
> Of a hundred, there lived but eight
> In thirteen hundred and forty-nine
> Of a hundred, there lived but nine.[4]

Or again, on one occasion the pope was informed by his advisers that the plague had killed 42,836,486 persons throughout the world and that German losses alone amounted to 1,244,434. Precision was not looked for in such matters; all that was meant to be conveyed was that the mortality had been fearful.

Later students varied widely in their determination of the plague's fourteenth-century mortality. Krafft-Ebing put the figure at three-fourths the entire population of Europe. Seebohm and Gasquet calculated that one-half the population of England died, a figure that Coulton placed nearer one-third. Hecker, the more conservative of the earlier scholars, decided that one-fourth of the population, or 25 million persons, had perished in

Europe. Using more sophisticated demographic devices, Élisabeth Carpentier studied the central Italian hill town of Orvieto and arrived at a mortality figure of 50 percent for the four months of plague in 1348. An equally thorough study was made of Prato, a town of some 6,000 persons, which revealed that about 25 percent had died in the plague sweep of 1630–1631. Even at 25 percent, the bubonic plague would remain the most catastrophic episode of disease ever recorded for Western Europe. The effects of such a monumental mortality can be examined from the viewpoint of economics, social institutions, the Church, war, and the general psychology of medieval man as revealed in his art and literature.

Contemporary Accounts

There are a number of chilling first-hand accounts of the plague. Best known among these is the introduction to the *Decameron*, the most famous work of the Florentine humanist, Giovanni Boccaccio (1313–1375). Indeed, it was flight from the plague by ten young men and women and the tales they told to pass the time that set the stage for the *Decameron*. Boccaccio wrote:

Not only did converse and consorting with the sick give the infection to the sound, but the mere touching of the clothes, or of whatsoever had been touched or used by the sick appeared of itself to communicate the malady. . . . A thing which had belonged to a man sick or dead of the sickness, being touched by an animal . . . in a brief time killed it . . . of this mine own eyes had experience. This tribulation struck such terror in the hearts of all . . . that brother forsook brother, uncle nephew, . . . often wife husband; nay (what is yet more extraordinary and well nigh incredible), some fathers and mothers refused to visit or tend their very children, as though they had not been theirs. . . . The common people, being altogether untended and unsuccored, sickened by the thousand daily, and died well nigh without recourse. Many breathed their last in the open street, whilst other many, for all they died in their houses, made it known to the neighbors that they were dead rather by the stench of their rotting bodies than otherwise; and of these and others who died the whole city was full. The neighbors, moved more by fear lest the corruption of the dead bodies should imperil themselves than by any charity for the departed, . . . brought the bodies forth from the houses and laid them before the doors where, especially in the morning, those who went about might see corpses without number. Then they fetched biers, and some, in default thereof, they laid upon a board; nor was it only one bier that carried two or three corpses, nor did this happen but once; nay, many might have been counted which contained husband and wife, two or three brothers, father and son, and the like. . . . The thing was come to such a pass that folk reckoned no more of men that died than nowadays they would of goats.[5]

Here we begin to sense the magnitude of the catastrophe and its effects on medieval thinking. It soon became apparent that the only hope for salvation lay in flight, a fact that helps explain why the mortality was higher among the poor, who simply lacked the wherewithal to flee and in any event had no place to go. Flight of the well-to-do also explains the near total dissolution of the social fabric that followed, because the wealthy included the rulers, religious leaders, and physicians, the very groups the citizenry ordinarily turns to when the social order is threatened by rampant disease.

Medicine was essentially impotent against the plague. Boccaccio wrote:

No doctor's advice, no medicine could overcome or alleviate this disease. An enormous number of ignorant men and women set up as doctors in addition to those who were trained. Either the disease was such that no treatment was possible or the doctors were so ignorant that they did not know what caused it, and consequently could not administer the proper remedy.[6]

Physicians themselves agreed with Boccaccio's grim pronouncement. Guy de Chauliac (1300–1368), the most famous French surgeon of the time, confessed that "the plague shamed the physicians, who could effect no cures at all, especially as, out of fear of infection, they dared not visit the sick."[7]

John of Burgundy wrote the most widely used tractate on prevention of the plague. His thought was copied by others and constituted much of the published medical advice to the populace. One such plagiarist was John Malverne, later physician to King Henry IV. After repeating much of the medical intelligence of John of Burgundy, Malverne's best advice was to flee any area in which plague was raging. Nor could the highest of churchmen escape the pervasive fear. According to one report, Pope Clement VI, who was then in Avignon, shut himself up and gave audience to no one.

None of this is meant to be judgmental. In truth, such behavior, even in community leaders, is easily comprehensible given the awful situation that existed and the all-too-obvious fact that the plague was not to be stayed by physicians or prayer. Certainly it must have appeared that virtue had disappeared from the earth. With all effective authority either gone or in disarray, a penitent period set in, but this was soon displaced by rampant immorality. The standards of society collapsed; the usual rules of behavior were abandoned; property rights forgotten; and a fatalistic hedonism became widespread.

The Plague and Economics

Obvious economic effects one might expect from a sudden large loss of human life are an increase in wages and a greater mobility of peasants, who at this point were locked to the lord's land and a fixed social status. There is evidence that both of these occurred. In certain instances, if laboring men could be found at all, they succeeded in obtaining increases of 50–100 percent in pay. Pressures also mounted for a redistribution of land. In England in July, 1348, the king noted that so many had died that the fields lay untilled. Due to a lack of demand, prices of agricultural products fell drastically.

In assessing the plague's overall impact, it must be remembered that epidemics were not limited to the years 1348–1350. The same pressures were renewed time and again. Between 1430 and 1480 major epidemics struck England on an average of once each four years, and the same pattern characterized plague on the Continent. From this it has been concluded that, demographically, the most important aspect of plague in fifteenth-century England was not the mortality of a given epidemic but the frequency of repeated epidemics. Under such relentless attack many landlords were forced to give their tenants domain over plots small enough to farm themselves, in exchange for cash rents. Each time the plague struck, another grain of sand in the mortar of the manorial system washed away. The argument that the plague was not a constant economic force is correct only because of the qualifier, constant. The point to be emphasized is that it was a recurrent economic force, and its accretions gradually changed the way men thought, which at times can be the most potent change of all. Even when the villein could not capitalize on his opportunity, he tasted a freedom he had never savored before. The peasant revolt of 1381 in England was symptomatic of a conjunction of forces. It is true that grievances had been accumulating during the first half of the fourteenth century, but these were bound to be accentuated by the economic exigencies occasioned by the mortality of the plague. The revisionist historians may be right in their discovery that in spite of many of the immediate social changes produced by the plague, the people largely reverted to their former situation within a few years after each epidemic. And it may also be true that by and large the rich became richer while the poor remained as they were. But something had changed, and that was the attitude between the two classes; a strong distrust was brought about that was inextricably bound up in the social change that finally took place.

Plague and the Church

Two characteristics of the Roman Catholic Church as it existed in the fourteenth century are germane to our story. First, it remained the single most influential force in the life of medieval man, and second, its hold was already weakening by the fourteenth century because of abuses of power now visible to anyone who cared to look. The plague debilitated the Church in a number of ways, all tied to the fact that it killed large numbers of clerics as well as members of the flock.

Many contemporary estimates of plague mortality among clerics can be found. Gasquet calculated that nearly half the clergy in England died between 1348 and 1350, a figure not changed much by later research. The bell tolled for the aristocracy of the Church as well as for parish priests. Of the 450 members of the pontifical court in Avignon, 94 died in 1348-1349. Of

28 cardinals alive in 1348, 9 died within the year. During the same period 25 of 64 archbishops and 207 of 375 bishops expired.

More recent commentators have demonstrated that the earlier figures of clerical mortality were too high. A number died of other causes, and many who were reported as vacating a benefice, and were thus assumed dead, had merely transferred or abandoned their ministry altogether. Even if we agree that the true number of plague deaths among beneficed clergy will never be known, there is no doubting that the loss was severe and that the effects were detrimental to the Church.

The ranks of churchmen were decimated at a time when the ravages of the plague called for more religious ministrations than ever before. The quality of those enlisted to fill the mounting vacancies is a disputed matter. On the one hand it has been argued that, because a surplus of parish priests existed in England at the time, most of the openings occasioned by the plague were filled with men already in priestly Orders. Others have contended that many positions had to be filled by quickly trained men and that even boys ten to fourteen years of age were taken on as oblates.

Setting aside the question of the quality of replacements, there is no doubt but that the Church lost influence as a result of the plague. Evidence for this comes from the highest halls of the Church itself. As the ordinary ecclesiastic joined the public in the increased avarice resulting from the plague, the mendicant orders, dedicated to surviving only by alms, emerged with heightened popular prestige. To head off this threat a petition was sent in 1351 by a group of higher churchmen to Pope Clement VI, urging a lesser role or even abolishment of the mendicant orders. The Pope's response is a telling indictment of the depths to which many clergymen had descended at the time.

And if their preaching be stopped [he asked], about what can you preach to the people? If on humility, you yourselves are the proudest of the world, arrogant and given to pomp. If on poverty, you are the most grasping and most covetous. . . . If on chastity – but we will be silent on this, for God knoweth what each man does and how many of you satisfy your lusts.[8]

In addition there was the basic question of the meaning and power of faith itself. In one view churchmen by this time had arrogated to themselves much more of God's power than Christ had ever intended. What did it mean then that priests and bishops were smitten by plague as readily as beggars and whores? Had they merely fallen from God's grace, which was ominous enough in itself, or could it be that prayer and faith counted for nothing in the affairs of man? What developed, then, was a new relationship between priest and laity. The parish was no longer a clerical manor; the divine powers of priests as well as landlords were now called into question.

Psychological Effects

No demographer can ever assess the psychological effects of the plague. To whatever imperfect extent this can be done, it must come from the recorded thoughts and actions of those who suffered the ordeal. By any measure the contemporary impact was profound, and the long-term effects pervasive and enduring. Some feeling for the immediate psychological perversions occasioned by the plague and the other natural disasters of the period can be found in the dancing mania, the emergence of the flagellants, and the persecution of the Jews. The more enduring psychological effects are reflected in the art and literature of the time.

The Dancing Mania

Episodes of what have been termed "dancing plagues" were known in Europe before 1347, but none included the large numbers of persons or the protracted fervor associated with those after the incursions by bubonic plague. The latter were known as the dances of St. John or more popularly St. Vitus. As recounted by "astonished contemporaries," the participants

formed circles hand in hand, and appearing to have lost all control over their senses, continued dancing, regardless of the bystanders, for hours together, in wild delirium, until at length they fell to the ground in a state of exhaustion. . . . While dancing they neither saw nor heard, being insensible to external impressions through the senses, but were haunted by visions, their fancies conjuring up spirits whose names they shrieked out; and some of them afterwards asserted that they felt as if they had been immersed in a stream of blood.[9]

The dancing mania spread from Germany to Aix-la-Chapelle in 1374, from there to the Netherlands and later to other cities in Europe, at times involving more than a thousand participants. A similar phenomenon appeared in Italy, where it was called tarantism and was thought to be due to the bite of a tarantula. The sufferers indulged in wild and protracted dancing and exhibited a large number of other symptoms which strike the modern reader as either feigned or hysterical. It was believed that music and dancing dispersed the tarantula's poison throughout the body and finally expelled it through the skin. Thus came into popularity the Tarantella, a sort of musical antidote to the spider's venom, which was played in different ways, depending on the moods observed in the victims. Tarantism did not peak in Italy until the seventeenth century, and of course the musical form survives today with few to appreciate its origins.

The Flagellants

As with the dancing mania the origins of the flagellant movement go back further than the plague period. Brotherhoods of the Church were dedicated to the penance of scourging as early as the eleventh century. In the beginning the flagellants were involved in a sort of surrogate penance. Their suffering was to atone for the sins of the populace and thereby remove the present danger or mollify the next. Gradually the townspeople joined in, rich and poor, high and low, marching through the street night and day, summer or winter, half-clothed, scourging themselves with leathern thongs until the blood flowed.

As with the dancing mania it was the plague that carried the flagellants to the extremes that finally turned church and secular authorities against them and effectively ended their influence. The extremist movement began in the fourteenth century with the emergence of the Brotherhood of the Flagellants in Hungary and spread first to Germany, then elsewhere in Europe. Gradually their assumed autonomy became a threat to the Church. The handwriting on the wall was clear after the Flagellants were denounced by a papal Bull in late 1349. From that point on the ecclesiastical campaign against them increased rapidly and the movement soon effectively died out.

Persecution of the Jews

The final persecution of the Flagellants, harsh though it was at times, was as nothing compared to the fate of European Jews. Before it was over, the anti-Semitic campaign of the plague years eclipsed in fury even that witnessed during the Crusades of the twelfth century. These prejudices had ancient origins which can only be sketched here. The basic alienation began with Jewish rejection of Christ as savior and the Gospels as a replacement for Mosaic law. St. Augustine reinforced the Christian position by labeling Jews as "outcasts." Their indictment as Christ-killers was formalized by Pope Innocent III in 1205, which led St. Thomas Aquinas to conclude that Jews were slaves of the Church. In the twelfth century the entire situation was inflamed by a growing belief that Jews were murdering Christians in a ritual repetition of the Crucifixion. Mixed in with such doctrinal matters was the issue of Jewish property. Simple greed cloaked in the guise of ideological outrage undoubtedly operated at times.

In such circumstances the plague arrived. Faced with a monstrous and mysterious mortality from the plague, and further terrified by the collapse of the usual social protections, the ignorant and superstitious mind demanded an explanation or, failing that, a scapegoat. Historically the latter role has been played by the Jews, although in the present instance, the Arabs of Spain and pilgrims in general also became targets of popular hostility.

The principal charge against the Jews was that they spread the plague by poisoning the public wells. In part this may have derived from the Jewish emphasis on basic hygiene, which led them to shun the frequently contaminated public wells and search for water from running streams. Such a practice could hardly escape notice in the general paranoia that followed the devastation of the plague.

The spark that started the conflagration of Jewish persecution throughout Europe in 1348-1349 was the confession, still extant, of a Jewish physician who, following a period on the rack, finally admitted spreading the plague. Thereafter the familiar and dismal slaughter spread from city to city. At times the massacre broke out while the plague was raging; at other times the approach of the epidemic into neighboring cities touched off the violence. A contemporary account places the total killed in Strasbourg alone at 16,000, probably an inflated figure, but tragic enough if halved. And so it went over Europe. At times the religious and secular leaders tried to contain the slaughter, at other times they incited it and even took part. By 1351 the plague had waned and with it went the Jewish persecution. There was really nothing unique about the attacks on Jews during the plague years except their extent and ferocity, which gave them no equal until the Nazi assaults of the twentieth century.

Death in Art

The effects of the plague and other medieval catastrophes were indelibly embedded in the art of central and southern Europe for more than three centuries after 1347. Death was at the center of this gloomy heritage, and as historians have shown, death was emphasized in the waning Middle Ages as never before or since. *Memento mori* was the byword of the age. But it was not death with redeeming qualities, death as an end to unhappiness or a deliverance from pain. It was death in all its gruesome glory, death as seen in the putrescent cadaver, death as the beautiful human being becoming a corpse, death as the stalker, ever ready to lay a bony hand on a fleeing shoulder. By now the fearful message of death's horror was not limited to the preacher's sermon; the woodcut had been invented to convey the morbid philosophy to the illiterate and faithless as well.

The most pervasive theme to come out of this period, a motif that would persist in art and literature for centuries, was the Dance of Death. Most commonly death appeared in the form of a skeleton, and when the invitation was extended, no one could refuse the dance. Knights and kings, priests and popes, peasants and physicians—all were susceptible to sudden oblivion, without regard to anything perceptible as justice.

The impartiality of death depicted repeatedly in the Dance of

Death was also a statement on the notion of social equality, as that concept was understood by medieval man. To the extent that this is true, it is a remarkable and further argument favoring the notion that changes in the medieval perception of the relationship between highborn and lowborn may have been a more important contribution of the plague than the changes that occurred in their institutions as such.

It is true that the gloomy art of the later Middle Ages had pre-plague origins, but after the travail of the fourteenth century, a basic change occurred; death had become an obsession. In part the increased emphasis on death in all its unredeeming aspects must have related to the death experienced vividly and often at the hands of epidemic diseases, principally bubonic plague.

Respite from War

One struggles to find a saving word to say on behalf of bubonic plague in fourteenth-century Europe. If there was any immediate human gain from the plague, it could have been in the arena of war. The kings of France and England, the Italian republics, and the Pope all had to discontinue their usual martial activities because of fear of the plague, loss of life among potential recruits, and diminishment of the revenue necessary to finance military activities. The two coalitions put together by Venice and Genoa were on the brink of war in 1345 but had to postpone hostilities until 1351. The civil war in Flanders began in 1346 but stopped when the plague rolled in two years later. One of Europe's most protracted conflicts, the Hundred Years' War, underwent a temporary truce because the plague had decimated the ranks of foot soldiers.

Though the respite from war was temporary, it was revealing. Any natural catastrophe that can hold war in abeyance, even temporarily, exerts a profound effect on the social structure at the time. True, the effects were not lasting; as soon as the plague permitted, men resumed their all-time-favorite outdoor sport. But history is not just a matter of change over centuries; it is told in terms of days and weeks as well, and for a brief span at least, the natural destruction of plague stilled man's deadly hand against his fellow man.

Summary

The total impact of the plague on the later Middle Ages has been variously assessed. At the one extreme are those who have singled out the epidemics of plague as marking the end of the medieval epoch, as events that almost produced a discontinuity in history. In these minds the repeated assaults of bubonic plague wiped out the immediately previous period of prosperity, altered political events, slowed military adventures, accelerated class struggles, accentuated nationalism, dictated artistic motifs, and precipitated aberrant behavior in the masses that can be characterized as psychological epidemics.

Others have concluded that the effects of the plague have been greatly exaggerated. They argue that in certain circumscribed areas, such as economics and population, the evidence has been misinterpreted altogether. These revisionists have relied on recent applications of demography to history, and while one may not argue with their findings that population and prosperity were already declining before the plague struck, one can reasonably dispute any extrapolation of such data to the conclusion that the plague had little or no effect. A problem with the demographic approach is that it looks at short, discrete episodes of time for explications of cause and effect. It is not enough, for example, to examine German social institutions in the preplague years of, say, 1330 and 1340 vis-à-vis the postplague year of 1350 and conclude that the observed effects were not all that profound. In the fourteenth century alone, plague returned to Germany in 1357–1362, 1370–1376, and 1380–1383. The same pattern marked Italy and, as we have seen, England. Epidemic diseases had visited Europe before 1348, but the recurrences exhibited by plague were new, and an accurate assessment of the plague's impact must take a correspondingly long-term view. The bare numbers of demography can reconstruct certain events in the Middle Ages, but they cannot reconstruct medieval life. That task, which can only be approximated at best, must call on all the tools of historiography, of which demography remains but one. Using the broader lens, the plague is seen as having had a genuine effect on European history, both at the time and for centuries thereafter. Medieval man has been called "a man on the defensive," and in part this was because of the plague.

All around him loomed inchoate shapes redolent with menace. Thunder crashed, lightning blazed, hail cascaded; evil forces were at work, bent on his destruction. He was no Siegfried, no Brunnhilde heroically to defy the elements. Rather, it was as if he had wandered in from another play: an Edgar crying plaintively, "Poor Tom's a-cold: poor Tom's a-cold!" and seeking what shelter he could against the elements.

Poor Tom survived, but he was never to be quite the same again.[10]

Can the Plague Return?

Is poor Tom finally secure against the cold? Have advances in medicine and public health removed industrialized societies from the threat of a future contagious epidemic of the magnitude of the plague in fourteenth-century Europe? The answer, as many would guess, is an unequivocal no. At any time the world can be visited by a plague-like pandemic, either from a new microorganism or from one of our older microscopic friends gone berserk.

Microbial mutations are occurring constantly. There is no reason why a new microorganism may not appear in our midst, one insensitive to all known antibiotics and for which no preventive vaccine can be developed in time to prevent a pandemic. Mutations are a natural form of recombining DNA, and already the process accounts for certain drug-resistant strains of gonococci and staphylococci. This is the process whereby we are periodically treated to a pandemic of influenza for which no vaccine is available, and indeed these epidemics alone are enough to demonstrate the possibility of a recurrence of 1348.

In fact our venerable nemesis, *Yersinia pestis,* has never really left us. Major outbreaks of bubonic plague occurred in London in 1665, France in 1720, Moscow in 1770, Yunnan in 1892, and Bombay in 1896. In 1900 a minor outbreak occurred in San Francisco's Chinatown and smoldered for several years. The ensuing events form an almost classical episode in the social history of disease. To protect the good name of San Francisco, city and state officials, including Governor Henry Gage, denied the existence of bubonic plague. They were joined by the press, by merchants who feared the economic impact, and even by physicians and the state board of health.

In the United States between 1900 and 1966, epizootics in urban rats caused a known 547 cases of human disease and 349 deaths. The population of ground squirrels, chipmunks, and prairie dogs in the Southwest harbors one of the larger reservoirs of plague bacilli in the world. There is nothing to prevent an urban outbreak at some future date. *Xenopsylla cheopis* is alive and thriving. *Rattus rattus* abounds in our cities, although its nocturnal habits and modern housing keep it out of the consciousness of all but our poorer citizens. And we are crowded together in the population clots that are necessary to close the deadly circle.

The Plague, by Albert Camus, is an allegorical representation of the Nazi occupation of France during World War II, but it provides genuine human insight into the psychology of a large city, isolated by quarantine, and confronted with bubonic plague. It also speaks to the question of the plague's return. In his book the disease finally burns itself out, and Camus ends in this way:

And indeed, as he listened to the cries of joy rising from the town, Doctor Rieux remembered that such joy is always imperiled. He knew what those jubilant crowds did not know but could have learned from books; that the plague bacillus never dies and disappears for good; that it can lie dormant for years and years in furniture and linen chests; that it bides its time in bedrooms, cellars, trunks, and bookshelves; and that perhaps the day would come when, for the bane and enlightening of men, it would rouse up its rats again and send them forth to die in a happy city.[11]

The principal shield protecting a modern American city from the return of diseases like bubonic plague is an intact social structure. Invoke any social catastrophe – a limited nuclear war will suffice – and bubonic plague can easily return for our "bane and enlightening." All that is needed is the collapse of our pharmaceutical industries, our system of public health, and our general governmental structure.

One major social change has occurred since 1348 that actually increases the likelihood of a pandemic, if pestilence should erupt in a technologically crippled world, and that is the speed of transportation. It will be recalled that the plague that raged in Sicily in 1347 did not reach Ireland until some eighteen months had elapsed. Principally this was because the plague could not spread any faster than the fastest human transport. Similarly, the cholera epidemic that originated in Bengal in 1826 did not reach the United States until 1832. By way of contrast, consider the particularly virulent outbreak of influenza in 1957. Within three to four months of its identification in Hong Kong, the virus was disseminated throughout the world, in large part due to the speed of modern transportation. The spread was so rapid that the largest pharmaceutical industry in the world could not produce vaccine in time to protect any but those considered the most deserving – old persons, pregnant women, and football players bound for the bowl games. Granted that influenza spreads by a different route than cholera, the point remains that the vastly beneficial effects of rapid transportation could, under certain circumstances, become a good deal less than benign.

The psychological effects bubonic plague had on medieval man have been considered. Chief among these were fear and panic, which were bad enough in 1348 but even quicker to rise in subsequent epidemics when people knew the plague's awful potential. Some believe that modern man, faced with bubonic plague, would react more rationally and restrainedly than medieval man, who suffered more because he was totally ignorant of the workings of the world, including any understanding of how the plague spread. The available evidence, however, does not support such a sanguine estimate of the favorable effects of education in the face of an epidemic, whether its cause is known or not. Yellow fever erupted in New Orleans in 1878 among people who believed that if they had been born and reared locally, they were immune to this particular affliction. When they saw their loved ones dying with the same symptoms as foreigners, a panic set in which was unprecedented in the history of epidemics in New Orleans. As the disease spread up the Mississippi, Memphis reacted in much the same way.

Or to consider the matter in strictly recent times, look at a few items culled from newspaper reports of the minor outbreak of cholera in Italy in 1973.

Health authorities told the Romans there was no reason for alarm, but hundreds flooded the only inoculation center in this city of 3 million people. . . . In one of Bari's poorest sections, residents harassed passengers in a car with Naples license plates; the people feared its occupants would spread the contagion.[12]

In San Giorgio, a rumor circulated that a man of 68 and his sister of 70 had come down with cholera, and more than 100 persons besieged their house shouting: "Take them away! Take them to the hospital!" The mob quieted down when a doctor examined the two old people and reported they had no sign of cholera. But the crowd's fears returned, and they piled old mattresses and furniture in the street and set them afire.[13]

Tens of thousands lined up at inoculation stations in and around Naples. . . . People came in and out of windows, smashing through glass panes. Police stepped in to stop violent quarrels among those waiting in line.[14]

This is an epidemic involving negligible mortality and morbidity in that most civilized of countries, Italy. In 1973.

Notes

1. Blum, J. M. *Woodrow Wilson and the Politics of Morality.* Boston: Little, Brown & Company, 1956, pp. 196-197.

2. Mather, C. *Magnolia Christi Americana,* vol. 1. Hartford, 1855, p. 55, quoted in O'Malley, C. D., ed. *The History of Medical Education.* Berkeley: University of California Press, 1970, p. 464.

3. Ell, S. "Interhuman Transmission of Medieval Plague," *Bull. Hist. Med.* 54:497-510, 1980.

4. Coulton, G. G. *The Black Death.* New York: Jonathan Cape & Harrison Smith, 1930, p. 49.

5. Boccaccio, G. *Tales from the Decameron,* translated by Richard Aldington. New York: Book League of America, 1930, pp. 2-5.

6. Ibid., p. 2.

7. De Chauliac, G. *La Grande Chirurgie.* Paris: Félix Alcan, 1890, p. 171.

8. Ziegler, P. *The Black Death.* New York: John Day Company, 1969, p. 267.

9. Hecker, J.F.C. *The Epidemics of the Middle Ages.* London: The Sydenham Society, 1846, pp. 87-88.

10. Ziegler, *Black Death.* P. 279.

11. Camus, A. *The Plague.* New York: Vintage Books, 1972, p. 287.

12. *Kansas City Star,* September 3, 1973, p. 1.

13. Ibid., September 10, 1973, p. 9.

14. Ibid., September 2, 1973, p. 11B.

Bibliographic Commentary

Earlier attempts at linking individual diseases to the course of history were inordinately simplistic and may have given the entire venture a bad name in the eyes of traditional historians. Examples of this genre are the two books by C. MacLaurin, *Post Mortem,* New York: George H. Doran, 1923; *Mere Mortals* by the same publisher in 1925; and J. A. Myers, *Fighters of Fate,* Baltimore: The Williams and Wilkins Company, 1925.

More recent and generally sounder, though not scholarly in the strict sense, are R. Marx, *The Health of the Presidents,* New York: G. P. Putnam's Sons, 1960; J. B. Moses and W. Cross, *Presidential Courage,* New York: W. W. Norton & Company, 1980; R. Stevenson, *Famous Illnesses in History,* London: Eyre & Spottiswoode, 1962; H. L'Etang, *The Pathology of Leadership,* New York: Hawthorn Books, 1970; F. R. Dumas, *Madness in Power,* Philadelphia: Chilton Book Company, 1969; and N. Fabricant, *Thirteen Famous Patients,* Philadelphia: Chilton Book Company, 1969.

Mercifully for all concerned, the earlier pretensions of psychohistory have been examined critically in recent years. The current surge of interest in the technique is usually dated to the presidential address delivered by William Langer to the American Historical Association in 1957 and published in the *Am. Hist. Rev.* 63:283–304, 1958. The deficiencies of the psychohistorical method as generally practiced were lucidly exposed by H. Trevor-Roper in his assessment of Walter Langer's book on Hitler which appeared in the *Sunday Times* (London), February 18, 1973, p. 35. A much more exhaustive treatment was presented by J. Barzun in the *Am. Hist. Rev.* 77:36–64, 1972. A fine recent overview is that by M. Shepherd, "Clio and Psyche: The Lessons of Psychohistory," *J. Roy. Soc. Med.* 71:406–412, 1978.

The neurological aspects of Wilson's case are derived mainly from E. A. Weinstein, "Woodrow Wilson's Neurological Illness," *J. Am. Hist.* 57:324–351, 1970. Also consulted were E. B. Wilson, *My Memoir,* New York: The Bobbs-Merrill Company, 1938; J. M. Blum, *Woodrow Wilson and the Politics of Morality,* Boston: Little, Brown & Company, 1956; J. D. Barber, *The Presidential Character,* Englewood Cliffs, N.J.: Prentice-Hall, 1977; A. S. Link, *Woodrow Wilson: Revolution, War and Peace,* Arlington Heights, Ill.: AHM Publishing Co., 1979; and E. A. Weinstein, *Woodrow Wilson: A Medical and Psychological Biography,* Princeton, N.J.: Princeton University Press, 1981.

Attempts at the large view of disease and history began with A. Hirsch, *Handbook of Geographical and Historical Pathology,* tr. by C. Creighton, London: The New Sydenham Society, 1883–1886, and H. Haeser, *Lehrbuch der Geschichte der Medicin und der epidemischen Krankheiten,* Jena: H. Dufft, 1875, and G. Fischer, 1881, 1882. Each of these occupied three volumes, and it is probable that the subject is now too extensive and complicated for any individual scholar.

Less ambitious but still meritorious efforts include A. Colnat, *Les epidémies et l'histoire,* Paris: Editions Hippocrate, 1937; W. R. Bett, *The History and Conquest of Common Diseases,* Norman: University of Oklahoma Press, 1954; E. H. Ackerknecht, *History and Geography of the Most Important Diseases,* New York: Hafner, 1965; F. Henschen, *The History and Geography of Disease,* New York: Delacorte Press, 1965; and A. W. Crosby, Jr., *The Columbian Exchange,* Westport, Conn.: Greenwood Press, 1975. W. H. McNeill, *Plagues and Peoples,* Garden City, N.Y.: Anchor Press/Doubleday, 1976, ventures into sheer speculation so often that it nearly destroys its useful aspects.

At least two bibliographies deserve mention: A. L. Bloomfield, *A Bibliography of Internal Medicine: Selected Diseases,* Chicago: University of Chicago Press, 1960, and E. H. Ackerknecht, "Causes and Pseudocauses in the History of Diseases," in L. Stevenson, ed., *A Celebration of Medical History,* Baltimore: Johns Hopkins University Press, 1982. The latter is particularly helpful in dealing with important individual diseases, including the noncontagious diseases, which have been generally neglected.

Though not primarily historical, a number of books by bacteriologists and epidemiologists are important to anyone working in the history of contagious diseases. Examples here are C. Nicolle, *Destin des maladies infectieuses,* Paris: F. Alcan, 1933; M. Greenwood, *Epidemics and Crowd Diseases,* New York: Macmillan, 1937; C.E.A. Winslow, *The Conquest of Epidemic Disease,* Princeton, N.J.: Princeton University Press, 1944; A. Cockburn, *Infectious Diseases,* Springfield, Ill.: Charles C. Thomas, 1967; and M. Burnet and D. O. White, *Natural History of Infectious Disease,* 4th ed., Cambridge: Cambridge University Press, 1972.

The story of scurvy and the settlement of California largely follows J. B. de C. M. Saunders, "Geography and Geopolitics in California Medicine," *Bull. Hist. Med.* 41:293-324, 1967. The plight of the Amerindians in the face of new diseases is covered by J. Duffy, *Epidemics in Colonial America,* Baton Rouge: Louisiana State University Press, 1953. Typhus and Napoleon have been recounted, albeit imperfectly, by E. Zinsser, *Rats, Lice and History,* Boston: Little, Brown & Company, 1935, and R. H. Major, *Disease and Destiny,* Lawrence: University of Kansas Press, 1958. Another aspect of this story which is usually ignored is covered by F. Prinzing, *Epidemics Resulting from Wars,* Oxford: Clarendon Press, 1916; and R. H. Moser, "Of Plagues and Pennants," *Military Review,* May, 1965, pp. 71-84.

The literature on bubonic plague is too vast to be fully recounted here. The usual starting points are J.F.C. Hecker, *The Epidemics of the Middle Ages,* London: The Sydenham Society, 1846; F. A. Gasquet, *The Great Pestilence,* London: Simpkin Marshall, Hamilton, Kent, & Co., 1893 (the second edition of the latter was reprinted in 1977 by AMS Press of New York, entitled *The Black Death of 1348 and 1349*); G. G. Coulton, *The Black Death,* New York: Jonathan Cape & Harrison Smith, 1930; and L. F. Hirst, *The Conquest of Plague,* Oxford: Clarendon Press, 1953. A more recent contribution is P. Ziegler, *The Black Death,* New York: John Day Company, 1969.

Regional treatments include C. F. Mullett, *The Bubonic Plague and England,* Lexington: University of Kentucky Press, 1956; J.F.D. Shrewsbury, *A History of Bubonic Plague in the British Isles,* Cambridge: Cambridge University Press, 1970; and his challenger, R. S. Gottfried, *Epidemic Disease in Fifteenth Century England: The Medical Response and the Demographic Consequences,* New Brunswick, N.J.: Rutgers University Press, 1978.

A monumental study of local accounts is J. N. Biraben, *Les Hommes et la peste en France et dans les pays européens et méditerranéens,* Paris: Mouton, 1975-1976. M. W. Dols, author of *The Black Death in the Middle East,* Princeton, N.J.: Princeton University Press, 1977; and J. Norris, author of "East or West? The Geographic Origin of the Black Death," *Bull. Hist. Med.* 51:1-24, 1977, debated the origin of bubonic plague to no ultimate resolution in "Geographical Origin of the Black Death," *Bull. Hist. Med.* 52:112-120, 1978.

John T. Alexander explores the Russian story in *Bubonic Plague in Early Modern Russia,* Baltimore: Johns Hopkins University Press, 1980. The resiliency of cultures assaulted by the plague in two small cities in Italy, Prato and Orvieto respectively, is revealed by C. M. Cippola, *Cristofano and the Plague,* Berkeley: University of California Press, 1973, and E. Carpentier, *Une ville devant la peste:*

Orvieto et la Peste Noire de 1348, Paris: SEVPEN, 1962.

The psychological aberrations associated with plague epidemics are discussed by Hecker and Ziegler (see above). The classic paper in this regard is G. Rosen, "Psychopathology in the Social Process. 2. Dance Frenzies, Demonic Possession, Revival Movements and Similar So-Called Psychic Epidemics," *Bull. Hist. Med.* 36:13–44, 1962. A recent treatment is that of B. W. Tuchman, *A Distant Mirror: The Calamitous Fourteenth Century*, New York: Alfred A. Knopf, 1978. The plague's effects on the arts are discussed in R. Crawfurd, *Plague and Pestilence in Literature and Art*, Oxford: Clarendon Press, 1914, and J. Huizinga, *The Waning of the Middle Ages*, Garden City, N.Y.: Doubleday Anchor Books, 1954.

Plague mortality among the clergy is examined by Shrewsbury (see above) and by B. J. Zaddach, *Die Folgen des schwarzen Todes für den Klerus Mittel-europas*, Stuttgart: G. Fischer, 1971.

The debate between traditionalists and revisionists, led in part by demographers, over the enduring effects of the plague is nicely summarized in W. M. Bowsky, ed., *The Black Death: A Turning Point in History?* New York: Holt, Rinehart & Winston, 1971.

3
DISEASE AS SUPERNATURAL

There is little that is obvious about the nature of disease. Even repeated close observations of illness at the bedside may yield no more accurate information about the true cause of disease than one learns about the solar system from watching the sun in its apparent east to west passage each day. In a raging epidemic of smallpox or bubonic plague, the essential sameness of the signs and symptoms may be discernible, and with experience, a certain amount of prognostication becomes possible. But the mere observation of such repetitious episodes of disease reveals nothing necessarily of what is being spread and how. The ultimate obscurity of disease is evidenced by the fact that even an assiduous application of the only two investigative tools humankind possessed for most of its history – observation and rationalization – could not elucidate the cause of a single important human disease until little more than a century ago. Excepting isolated situations, as we shall see, the management of disease through specific therapy and prevention likewise were twentieth-century accomplishments. These facts, at times surprising to the beginning student of disease, are more comprehensible to those who are familiar with the complexities of the human body and the disruptions of structure and function we term disease.

There are insurmountable limitations to understanding disease by simple observation. Fever, for instance, is a frequent and

easily detectable finding in which the initial symptoms and signs
are often identical regardless of the cause. Yet in a case of yellow
fever, death may result, while with influenza the fever may last
three days then disappear. The pain of appendicitis characteristically localizes immediately over the inflamed organ, so much so
that the site bears a name, McBurney's point. Yet, in certain instances, the appendix is naturally situated behind that portion of
the large intestine from which it derives. In this situation the infected appendix does not contact the inner layer of the abdominal wall, and the characteristic pain and tenderness may be ab-
sent. Even more misleading is what is called referred pain. The
dolor of the heart condition known as angina pectoris may be
limited to the left arm, that of a ureteral stone to the testicle, that
of pneumonia in the lower lung to the shoulder, that of gall bladder disease to a point under the right scapula.

The natural course of disease can be equally deceiving. Apparently minor mishaps can lead to death, while clearly frightening
episodes of illness may prove harmless. Picking up a thorn in the
foot, so innocuous that the episode may be forgotten, can lead to
the convulsive death of tetanus two weeks later. Yet the equally
awesome convulsions of epilepsy leave a sufferer apparently
none the worse for the experience. The grand mal seizure of epilepsy is, in fact, particularly useful in demonstrating the obscurity of disease. A strapping young warrior, to all appearances a
paradigm of good health, suddenly emits an eerie cry, falls to the
ground, chews blood from his tongue, loses control of bowels
and bladder, and suffers ten minutes of bone-jarring convulsions. He then falls asleep for an hour or two and awakens, not
only unharmed but unable to recall anything related to the
event.

No inspired insight is needed to understand why the supernatural approach to diseases arose, became as pervasive as it did,
and persists even today. Supernatural belief provides the solace
of explanation when the human mind cannot understand the
nature of disease, or control its course, or find any appreciable
justice in the pattern of those afflicted. Look again on poor Job,
smitten with "sore boils from the sole of his foot unto his crown."
Granted, he was not a perfect man; still, many about him were
demonstrably as evil and yet escaped Satan's awful ministrations. Where is the sense in it all? What is the nature of the sores

and why are they so refractory to healing? The utter helplessness of man in the face of disease demands explanation, and that explanation has been found more often in supernatural than rational concepts. Or reconsider the warrior with epilepsy. The human mind, at least insofar as we understand its workings, simply could not witness such a spectacle without concocting an explanation. Even today the clonic fury of a grand mal seizure can shake the professional composure of students of medicine and nursing. In its instantaneous onset, awesome violence, and quick recovery, the seizure practically decrees a supernatural explanation. Look even at the word medical usage has assigned the phenomenon — *seizure*. And since there is no apparent natural force capable of seizing, a resort to the supernatural becomes all but rational under the circumstances.

In terms of numbers of persons, disease viewed as supernatural has easily been the dominant conception in human history. This is true of Europe and America as well as Asia and Africa. Further, as we shall see, elements of disease-as-supernatural remain to varying degrees even in those countries where scientific medicine has reached its highest development.

Prehistoric Disease

Before approaching the supernatural conception of disease, it remains to examine briefly the problem of studying prehistoric disease. Ideally, a comprehensive conceptual history of disease would begin with disease in the prehistoric period. The problem here, of course, is implicit in the definition of prehistory, that is, the period for which we have no written record. The study of concepts in the absence of written records might be likened to the study of paleontology without fossils. This inherent limitation leaves two possible alternatives. We can limit our attempt at understanding prehistoric disease to a few pictures on the walls of caves plus what we can learn from paleopathology, the study of the tracks disease has left in bones, teeth, fossils, and the like. Or we can study disease as it is conceived by primitive peoples and assume that their conceptions are the same as, or similar to, the way disease was perceived by prehistoric human beings. Each approach has its weakness. The study of paleopathology can tell us something of the types of disease that afflicted prehistoric persons, but little of what they thought about their ailments. On the other hand, equating primitive thinking about disease with that of prehistoric peoples becomes ultimately a matter of faith; it is at bottom an unprovable hypothesis.

The solution adopted in this book, as it has been in others, is dictated by desperation, that is, to take the best of both approaches and acknowledge the result as something less than perfect. We thus take the conceptually impoverished offerings of paleopathology and add an examination of primitive concepts of disease, to erect the best *possible* explanation of disease as it existed among our prehistoric ancestors, with the repeated reminder that the product is a description of a probability and nothing more.

From paleopathologists we learn that prehistoric persons suffered at least some of the same diseases we recognize today. With varying degrees of certainty, bony remains have identified prehistoric tuberculosis, syphilis, leprosy, tumors, rickets (deficiency of vitamin D), yaws, kidney stones, arthritis, and, of course, trauma. Incidentally, one scholar attempted to prove the existence of prehistoric bonesetters by a study that demonstrated a remarkable degree of healing in over 50 percent of the fractured bones he examined. The force of his conclusion was weakened by a study that showed similar healing in 36 percent of fractures examined in bones of wild gibbons. The conclusion was that the human fractures, like those of the gibbons, healed spontaneously. One presumably tongue-in-cheek scientist beclouded the issue further by asking if the recent discovery that chimpanzees utilize tools should raise the possibility that gibbons may function as orthopedists.

A major limitation of paleopathology is that it must depend on those human structures which have survived the millennia of human existence. This excludes the soft tissues, the brain, lung, heart, liver, intestines, and kidneys, those organs wherein most fatal and disabling disease occurs. A few fossilized bacteria have survived a million years or more, but organs of the prehistoric human body have not survived to help the paleopathologist in his task.

Although technically no longer in the realm of prehistory, pathological examinations were carried out in some eight thousand Egyptian mummies when the first Aswan dam was under construction. Unfortunately these were not meticulously done and the information they provided was scanty. More recent and careful examinations have been carried out on an Egyptian mummy and an ancient Chinese woman. The latter proved to have arteriosclerotic involvement in her coronary arteries, disproving the notion that this ailment depends exclusively on the stress of modern living, or more likely, suggesting that the stress of living is not uniquely modern. On one of the recent mummy autopsies, electron microscopy was demonstrated as feasible. The principal drawback, then, is not technology, but the dearth of available mummies, and we have seen that an even greater void exists for the prehistoric period proper.

Primitive Concepts of Disease

Turning our attention to the analogy between prehistoric and primitive concepts of disease causation, we find that the latter are susceptible to a variety of classifications, all of which contain a certain amount of overlapping.

The first is that sickness can be caused by sorcery, that is, by human beings accomplished in magic or able to exert a measure of control over supernatural events. Sorcerers operate either by creating a small image of the victim and abusing it (imitative) or by magical manipulation of a discarded part of the victim such as hair, nail clippings, or excrement (contagious).

A second primitive concept of disease causation is the breaching of taboo, in which disease emanates from the gods as punishment for either conscious or unconscious rupture of religious or social prohibitions.

A third concept, perhaps the oldest of all primitive notions of disease causation, is object intrusion. This may result from intrusion of any one of many objects, such as pebbles, splinters, or bits of bone or hair, into the victim's body by magical means. The objects are always tangible, although not usually pathogenic in our sense of the word.

Fourth, in addition to intrusion of material objects, disease can result from spiritual presence. In this system the victim falls ill because he has been invaded by an evil spirit or demon.

Fifth, disease can result from loss of soul. This can come about either by magical intervention during sleep or by abduction of the soul by ghosts or sorcerers during wakefulness.

In addition to the magical and religious conceptions, certain primitives at times look at disease in a way that can be termed natural, that is, an arising apart from human or divine intervention. In general these conditions are less important to our story, because they involve minor ailments that might better be termed discomforts than diseases. On Eddystone Island the natives spoke of these conditions as "coming of themselves," an opinion expressed by natives throughout Melanesia. Because the ailments are minor, they do not stimulate a search for causes. When they demand treatment, the medicine man may utilize the same modalities he uses against the more serious diseases.

Almost universally, in primitive as well as industrialized societies, some individual or group emerges to fill the role of healer. In primitive settings this individual has been variously called leech, shaman, and medicine man, and his function varied widely from tribe to tribe. Whatever his name, his role was often far more than that of mere healer. He was responsible for the entire tribal welfare, from control of the weather to ensuring a bountiful harvest to bringing about a favorable outcome in battle with enemy tribes. He was far more important to his society than his modern counterpart.

The medicine man utilized both religion and magic. In truth, in a given practice it is often impossible to sort out the two. For our purposes there is little reason to try; the medicine man himself would have made no such distinction, nor indeed would he have understood why he should try.

Primitive Therapeutics

Returning to the five categories of disease causation developed earlier, we find therapeutics to be simple and relatively straightforward. Sorcery is treated by countermagic which either neutralizes or overpowers the offending magic. Breach of taboo is managed by confession or by propitiating the gods. Disease-object intrusion is cured by removal of the object, often by sucking, a feat requiring a highly developed sleight-of-hand. Spirit intrusion is treated by one or more of three methods: incantations or invocation of more powerful demons; driving out the spirit by mechanical means such as loud noises, bleeding, or ingestion of preparations of noxious herbs; or by entangling the invading spirit in a special bundle of twigs passed gently over the patient's body. Loss of soul is countered by restoring the soul by a variety of means.

Primitive systems of medical belief are not as irrational as they appear at first glance. Indeed, excepting the initial premise, they are generally as logical as our own. For the Western rationalist, who, in search of understanding, can take the first step in the primitive scheme, the rest of the walk comes easily. For example, there is a Western Congo fetish for protection against sore throat, one version of which is a small doll with a reflecting device at the site of the umbilicus. The key to the protective function of this particular fetish is the notion that the demon of sore throat is terrifyingly ugly. When he comes near a home which is protected by the appropriate fetish, the demon sees his reflection and flees his own fearful visage. If the premise is accepted, if you believe that sore throat is caused by an ugly demon, the preventive practice itself becomes thoroughly rational.

Empiricism and Trephination

In their approach to therapy, in addition to religion and magic, primitive medicine men utilized a form of what I will term empiricism. The term empiricism can be troublesome to readers encountering its use in medical history for the first time. One definition of an empiric is charlatan or quack. Another relates to a group of Greek physicians that existed in Alexandria about the end of the third century B.C. This school of medical thought eschewed all theorizing and scientific experimentation in favor of experience alone, thus their title, Empiricists. As used here to describe the third early approach to managing disease, empiricism weds the ideas of experimentation and experience in a crude form of trial and error; the practices were crude in that no attempt was made to control the many variables. A new herb or mineral or surgical procedure was tried in a given episode of illness. If patients appeared to improve with some consistency, the new modality was added to the physician's armamentarium. If the results were sufficiently dire, the agent was abandoned. Empiricism in this sense was important to prehistoric man in more than medical ways; it was the process whereby he came to know his environment – what he could eat without causing illness, what he could touch without causing painful rashes, which snakes he could handle, and so on.

There is no reason why prehistoric man, through trial and error, should not have adopted naturally occurring substances to succor the sick as well as to dispatch his enemies. Certainly history has recorded many such events among peoples using nothing but crude empiricism. Opium for the control of pain is probably mentioned in the Ebers papyrus, which describes Egyptian therapeutics of around 1500 B.C. Recent work has demonstrated that the honey employed in the treatment of wounds by these same Egyptians has definite antibacterial action. Rauwolfia was used as a sedative for centuries in India before Western physicians in the 1950s began using its active substance, reserpine, in the treatment of high blood pressure. Other examples of the fruits of this form of empiricism are discussed in the chapter on specific therapy.

Dividing the primitive approach to disease into magical, religious, and empirico-rational is a useful analytic artifice but often does not describe the reality of a given conception of disease. The practice of trephination can be helpful in demonstrating the difficulties inherent in sorting out the conceptions responsible for a given medical practice. Trephination is an operation that opens a hole in the skull. Variously it has been accomplished by cutting, scraping, or punching a series of smaller holes, then cutting the bridges between them. The practice has been extremely widespread both temporally and geographically. Trephined skulls have been identified as far back as the Neolithic period, and the practice persists today in certain tribes of the South Pacific. The skulls have been found in France, Spain, Portugal, Algiers, Austria, Sweden, Belgium, Poland, and Russia and in North and South America, primarily in Peru and Mexico but also in Argentina and Canada.

When these skulls were first brought to light, historians were understandably incredulous. The fibrous coverings of the brain, the meninges, are extremely susceptible to infection by a number of microorganisms, producing meningitis, a disease dreaded even in our era of antibiotics. Why would prehistoric and primitive peoples undertake such a dangerous operation? This question has been asked many times by medical historians, anthropologists, and others, but a final answer eludes us. The consensus, if there is one, seems to be that the practice existed for religious, magical, and at times perhaps even medical reasons. Evidence for the involvement of religion and magic derives from the fact that trephination was practiced on dead as well as living subjects. Further, the round or oval pieces of bone removed, now termed *rondelles,* were often worn around the neck as amulets. (Amulets are devices for warding off evil, as opposed to talismans, which are supposed to bring good fortune.)

Medical motives for trephination may have existed as well. It is altogether possible that some medicine man, in the process of trephining to remove the evil spirit of headache, may have happened on a large blood clot or benign tumor and thereby saved his patient's life. Achieving the right result for the wrong reason is far from uncommon in the history of therapy, or in science generally for that matter. Despite the harrowing nature of trephination, survival was not a rarity. Proof of this comes from the large number of skulls in which the edges of the bony incision show evidence of new growth. In one study of 214 Peruvian skulls, complete healing was deemed present in over 55 percent, and early healing in another 16 percent. One specimen exists in which the operation was performed seven times.

Hebrew Medicine – Rational or Religious?

In the end, the enigma of trephination defies complete resolution. It thus characterizes a common problem in the earlier periods of the history of disease: How does one sort out religious and magical motivation from practices that today appear to have been sound hygiene or therapy? Certain practices of the ancient Hebrews as described in Leviticus 13–18 appear to have been remarkably prescient in light of current understanding. Indeed, the ancient Hebrews have been termed the founders of preventive medicine. If this means that their priests enforced the conception of cleanliness, which was highly valued by the Hebrews and surrounding groups before them, and that this enforced cleanliness produced more or less inadvertent hygienic practices, well and good. If it is meant to imply that the Hebrew priests knew that their actions were preventing specific diseases, then the matter is far less certain. The following example illustrates the contradictory nature of the Biblical evidence.

Hebrew priests were charged with examining homes of lepers to determine if they were still infected. The priest entered the house, and if "the disease is in the walls of the house with greenish or reddish spots, and if it appears to be deeper than the surface," the priest was to leave and close up the house for seven days. Leprosy today is very difficult to contract by person-to-person contact, but the leprosy of Biblical times may have been a good deal more infectious. Whether leprosy could have been contracted from the inanimate objects of a house is itself doubtful, but even if isolation helped, problems of interpretation remain. The spots and the seven-day quarantine simply make no sense in terms of what we now know about leprosy.

On the other hand, in Leviticus 13:45 the priests ordained that the "leper who has the disease shall wear torn clothes and let the hair of his head hang loose, and he shall cover his upper lip and cry, 'Unclean, unclean.' He shall remain unclean as long as he has the disease; he is unclean; he shall dwell alone in a habitation outside the camp." The practice of isolation as described here would have been reasonable in dealing with a more virulent and contagious disease than leprosy now is. The problem remains insoluble in part because the precise method by which leprosy spreads is still not known. Attempts at infecting human volunteers have uniformly failed, and indeed no animal could be made to harbor the disease until the armadillo and a species of monkey acquiesced in very recent times.

At first glance the Hebrews appear to have recognized the genetic dangers of consanguineous marriage to which their long history of inbreeding had rendered them susceptible. But when one examines their laws governing sexual intercourse, inconsistencies again arise. Sexual liaison was prohibited with one's father, mother, brother, sister, aunt, and uncle, all of which make sense in terms of preventing genetic disease. But also outlawed was intercourse with one's daughter-in-law, brother's

wife, daughter of a woman with whom you have also had intercourse, wife's sister if wife is still alive, and one's neighbor's
wife. This forces us to the conclusion that the strictures as a
whole were adopted for social rather than medical purposes. The
Hebrews were essentially tribal peoples at this time, and in the
interest of social tranquillity, strict rules governing the choice of
sexual partners were necessary. Intercourse was further prohibited with menstruating women, in keeping with the conception
of cleanliness, and between man and man or man and beast,
where the restriction is almost certainly moral.

Egyptian Medicine

Other ancient civilizations which influenced Western conceptions of disease were those of the Assyrians and the Egyptians.
To treat these two great epochs in a paragraph or two in a general history of medicine would clearly be a travesty. But in a conceptual history of disease, just such a cavalier treatment
becomes possible because Assyrian and Egyptian medicine featured the same three basic concepts already discussed – magic,
religion, and empirico-rationalism. Granted that there exist
many differences of emphasis in belief and practices, the conceptual core remains the same in its essential features.

One facet of Egyptian medicine that can serve our purpose
here is known from one of their medical papyri that differs from
the others. When it comes to therapy, most papyri are filled with
magic and religion. The Ebers Papyrus (ca. 1500 B.C.), while it
shows that the Egyptians recognized specific diseases and attempted clinical descriptions of such conditions as arthritis and
worm infestation, remains essentially magical in its approach to
treatment. It begins with several incantations against disease and
includes some 875 recipes such as the following:

Another for *blindness:* pig's eyes, its humour is fetched, real stibium, red
ochre, less of honey, are ground fine, mixed together, and poured into
the ear of the man, so that he may be cured immediately. Do [it] and
thou shalt see. Really excellent! Thou shalt recite as a spell: I have
brought this which was applied to the seat of yonder trouble: it will
remove the horrible suffering. Twice.[1]

Contrast this with the Smith Papyrus (ca. 1600 B.C.), which is given over to a discussion of forty-eight cases of clinical surgery. One case describes the method for reducing a dislocation of the mandible, the movable bone of the face.

If thou examinest a man having a dislocation in his mandible, shouldst thou find his mouth open [and] his mouth can not close for him, thou shouldst put thy thumb[s] upon the ends of the two rami of the mandible in the inside of his mouth, [and] thy two claws [meaning two groups of fingers] under his chin, [and] thou shouldst cause them to fall back so that they rest in their places. Thou shouldst say concerning him "one having a dislocation in his mandible. An ailment which I will treat."[2]

To this remarkably modern-sounding description, today's physician would add only the insertion between the teeth of a small roll of gauze or tape so that when the dislocated bone slipped back into its proper joint, the powerful masseter muscles would not snap the jaw shut leaving thy thumbs behind the patient's teeth.

The Smith Papyrus is singled out for two contributions it makes to the conceptual story of disease. First, it reveals an emphasis on empiricism and rationalization that surpasses anything we have seen to date or indeed will find until we consider Greek medicine of the period 400 B.C. and afterward. The procedure for reducing a dislocated mandible and other directions listed in the Smith Papyrus could only have derived from repeated meticulous observations of similar cases, and the treatment recommended could have been fixed on as superior to other methods only after numerous instances of trial and error.

The second conceptual message offered by the Smith Papyrus relates to the fact that it is superior to the nonsurgical papyri in terms of our perception of the useful information these documents contain. In a later chapter we will learn that the appearance of modern medicine coincided with a conceptual shift from the idea of disease as generalized to the view that held disease to be localized in origin. For much of Western history physicians and surgeons constituted two wholly different professional classes. Physicians were educated persons of relatively high social status, while surgeons were illiterate and of distinctly lower caste. As we will see, throughout its history the very

nature of surgery predisposed to localistic thinking. Gangrene of
the foot or hand automatically suggests a localized solution,
amputation. Because surgeons naturally thought in localistic
terms both in diagnosis and treatment, they remained relatively
immune to the theorization that had to be employed by physicians dealing with the obscure internal diseases. Thus unencum-
bered, surgeons in their interventions probably accomplished
more genuine healing than was possible for the socially and
educationally superior physicians. The Smith Papyrus shows us
that the practical advantages of thinking in localized terms were
present all along. As the story unfolds, however, it turns out that
these advantages were not perceived by physicians in general
until the nineteenth century, some 3,500 years after the extant
Smith Papyrus was composed.

Supernaturalism and Physicians

Perhaps the most remarkable aspect of the history of disease as
supernatural is the degree to which physicians managed to separate themselves from the notion that their patients were sick
because they had sinned. The evidence in the oldest texts from
Egypt and Mesopotamia does not permit a judgment on the matter, but in some Hippocratic writings (ca. 400 B.C.), it is clear that
disease was viewed as natural. Even in the Middle Ages and
Renaissance, when, in part due to the all-powerful influence of
Roman Catholicism, sin was held responsible for disease, physicians by and large remained free to think of disease as natural. If
ever a disease invited divine explanation it was syphilis, with its
moral implications of *coitus impurus*. Yet, among others, the sixteenth-century humanist Ulrich von Hutten ridiculed the notion
of syphilis as sin, maintaining that Nature's innate powers of producing change could result in new diseases as well.

The physician's affinity for a natural explanation of disease in
the face of prevailing Church dogma was not altogether a matter
of courage. In part, physicians, in the hierarchy that came to exist, were not obligated to deal with soul. They were students of
natural philosophy, which, while lower in rank than theology,
was a legitimate area of intellectual endeavor. They were not ex-

pected to be versed in theology, but were expected to restrict their efforts to bodily disease and avoid the assignment of moral guilt. By the time of Elizabethan England physicians, for practical purposes, had completely separated themselves from supernatural causation. One finds an occasional pious reference in the prefaces to medical texts of this time, but scant mention of supernatural elements thereafter. At the same time, however, their recipes for cure frequently contained the convenient caveat that they would work only if God so willed.

But if physicians managed a more or less complete theoretical separation between formal religion and disease, in practice they never abandoned the power of faith. And this went beyond merely exhorting a seriously ill patient to draw on whatever inner strength he or she could muster from personal religious convictions. It may be a matter of some embarrassment to those medical practitioners who would rather their art be purely scientific, but faith remains a strong feature in current medical practice. Even in scientific literature, one finds medicine dealing with religion and magic, as in case reports of stigmata (bleeding into the skin that is not self-induced) and hexing as a cause of regional enteritis (inflammation of the small intestine). The use of placebos (imitation medicines or procedures), although widely used for centuries, depends largely on the patient's belief (faith) that the medical agent has the power to allay the symptoms or eliminate the disease. Formerly thought to be physiologically inert, it now appears that placebos not only look like medication but actually produce measurable physiological responses. This fact greatly complicates the problem of testing the efficacy of new drugs and procedures, such as laetrile in treating cancer or acupuncture for surgical anesthesia.

In one sense medical professionals have not so much abandoned as transferred the object of faith from religion to medicine, at times even to themselves. The diplomas and certificates on the office wall are reminiscent of the votive offering from grateful patients that adorned the walls of healing temples in ancient Greece. Where the shaman wears a costume associated with healing in the minds of his clients, the modern physician dons a white coat, the stethoscope around the neck, or if in the coat pocket, arranged so that one earpiece is discreetly visible.

Where the medicine man rattled his bladder full of bones, his modern counterpart writes out a prescription with strange symbols and folds it carefully before handing it to his patient. All of this is designed to enhance the mystical image of healing power and thus increase the likelihood that the patient will feel better for the encounter. The reflective physician does not resist the power of faith, nor shamefully neglect his magical aura, but accepts it as a useful element now as it has always been in the past.

Modern Faith Healing

The use of faith in healing has had a far more visible and uninterrupted existence in the nonmedical setting than within the healing professions. Today, if anything, it has a large and growing following. In person or by radio and television, thousands of Americans seek the succor of mystical healers such as Kathryn Kuhlman and Oral Roberts. Before he died in 1971 in an automobile accident, the Brazilian peasant Arigó was seeing as many as 300 patients daily, diagnosing and treating in a matter of minutes, frequently performing minor surgery on the spot with a pocketknife.

The greatest healing shrine in the West is at Lourdes, France, which had its beginning with the famous visions of Bernadette Soubirous in 1858. The process of healing as it has evolved at Lourdes is so perfectly designed to accomplish its aim – the enhancement of faith in the divine cure of illness – that it merits some detailing. Beginning with the decision to make the pilgrimage, everything that happens is designed to increase the expectation and confidence of cure. Money is raised, often as a community effort or from family contributions. Local masses are offered. Members of the family and even the patient's priest or physician make the trip, thereby underscoring the wide hopes and support available to the patient. Once at Lourdes the sick person is among a sea of pilgrims who have traveled from all over the world for the same purpose and with the same conviction that something salutary is about to happen. The days are occupied with prayer and trips to the Grotto, where the supplicant is immersed in the icy spring. Each afternoon the pilgrims, usually forty to fifty thousand, assemble at the Esplanade for the climax of the day's activities, during which the religious fervor is carefully orchestrated to a crescendo in which all voices in a crowd extending as far as the eye can reach are raised in prayer for relief of the afflicted. If faith can contribute to healing, it should not surprise us to find abandoned crutches and wheel-chairs in the environs of Lourdes.

At least one organized Western religion, Christian Science, operates on the belief that disease has no reality. Its founder was Mary Baker Eddy, who held its first public service in Lynn, Massachusetts, on June 6, 1875. The Church of Christ, Scientist, as it is properly known, was formally chartered in 1879. Some intimation of the domestic difficulties life dealt Mrs. Eddy can be found in the names she accrued in her several marriages, becom-ing finally Mary Morse Baker Glover Patterson Eddy. Through-out her life she suffered a variety of pains and illnesses, at times leading to dependence on morphine. In 1862 she was treated by one Phineas Parkhurst Quimby, a clockmaker by trade, but more important to us as a traveling mesmerist who later dropped hypnotism in healing because of a conviction that disease was merely "an error of the mind." Quimby met great success as a healer, and it was this reputation that took Mrs. Eddy to him in Portland, Maine, in 1862. Very shortly she was well. Four years later she suffered the bittersweet fall on the ice which led to the formation of Christian Science. Three days after sustaining this injury to her back, she read the words of Matthew 9:2 and left her bed, ostensibly healed.

As time passed Mrs. Eddy preferred to discount Quimby's influence and attributed her success to a direct revelation from God. Despite the success of her mission, her later years were filled with physical suffering. Frequent attacks of kidney stones drove her back to morphine, and she lived in constant fear of the malicious animal magnetism, the destructive mental telepathy, which she held responsible for the personal misfortunes she began suffering in the 1870s. Despite her many physical ail-ments she survived until 1910 and age eighty-nine.

In 1932 Mrs. Eddy was reviled by Morris Fishbein, the fore-most spokesman of organized medicine in the United States, as a fraud, a charlatan, and plagiarist. Such attacks had little impact on the success of the movement. Federal census figures revealed a United States membership of 85,717 in 1906, 202,098 in 1926, and 268,915 in 1936. Such figures are no longer available, but the number of Christian Science churches in the United States alone approximated 2,400 in 1977. The larger importance of Christian Science is not its rapid early growth nor its durability, but its demonstration that large numbers of Americans were developing a new form of religious emphasis, the heart of which was the conviction that faith can heal.

If faith healing is as alive as ever, so are its excesses. According to press reports, in Würzburg, the city where some 300 witches were burned for trafficking with the devil in one year in the seventeenth century, a young girl died in 1976 of malnutrition and dehydration following ten months of exorcism by two priests. In Barstow, California, in 1973, one enthusiast became so convinced that religious ministrations had cured his diabetes that he threw away his insulin, only to die within days as his family stood by. In Cortez, Colorado, in 1974, a four-year-old died of diphtheria after her family refused medical help on religious grounds. The family believed that earthly life was of little consequence compared to the judgment of God thereafter. As with the natives who use a fetish to scare off the demon of sore throat, if you accept the basic premise of faith healing, everything that follows appears rational.

In a very real sense all therapy is empirical. Every time a patient receives a drug for the first time – even an old, well-established drug – an experiment takes place. This is true because our physiologies as well as our personalities are individual. The same dose of the same drug may be absorbed at a different rate in two individuals, but even if absorption is identical, the effects may be altogether different. A five-grain aspirin tablet can relieve a headache in one person and produce a sudden asthmatic death in another. The reasons for these differences are still largely unknown, but the effect is that new drugs derived by scientific or controlled empiricism revert to the cruder form of trial and error when they are given to individuals for the first time.

Controlled empiricism is a recent development in the history of therapeutics. The aim of scientific empiricism is to be certain that the effects observed after a given therapy is administered are due to the agent itself. This is far more difficult than many would suppose. The most sophisticated new approach is the double blind experiment and its variations, in which neither the experimenter nor the subject know whether the therapeutic agent is genuine or sham.

For most of history, no such elaborate precautions were taken. Almost all of the drugs and procedures employed before the twentieth century were developed by empiric methods not unlike those described for primitive peoples, in short, simple trial and error. Indeed, most of the drugs in use today were adopted by physicians before anyone knew how they worked. A severely attenuated list would include aspirin for fever, digitalis for heart failure, cortisone for arthritis, barbiturates and tranquilizers for sedation, reserpine for high blood pressure, phenothiazines for schizophrenia, lithium for the manic phase of manic-depressive illness, and morphine for pain.

The primitive view of disease and the actions taken to combat it have been surveyed briefly. The contention has been that all of the elements of primitive medicine are visible on the current scene and that at times they remain useful even to the so-called scientific physician. If the matter were left at this point, an unbalanced picture would result, because there are profound drawbacks to the primitive approach to disease. As long as one views disease causation as supernatural, the possibility of meaningful human intervention is limited. Little understanding of anatomy, physiology, or biochemistry will accrue with such a model of illness because it eliminates the need for such understanding. One historian brought together the small group of available primitive autopsies which had been performed to try to discover the cause of death, and concluded that the exercises contributed nothing to the understanding of the human body or to disease causation as we use the term. This finding is easily understood. Ordinarily, we take from a scientific investigation only the answers to the questions we have posed. Thus it is not surprising to find that the rare primitive dissector gleaned different information from his autopsy than would a modern pathologist. For the primitive, perfectly normal organs might be interpreted as pathological. We will revisit this phenomenon when we encounter Renaissance anatomists who paid scant attention to organs deformed by disease because they were trying to discover normal anatomy, and because in any event they did not conceive of disease as localized.

For the same reasons, the medicine man has scant use for clinical medicine, that is, repeated close observation of diseases at the bedside. His system of belief does not demand that diseases be named and classified. He may use the elements of clinical medicine in a rudimentary form, but his theory is applied without a conception of specific diseases as we know them. The need for anatomical and physiological knowledge and for close clinical observation arises only if disease is perceived as natural in its origin and course, a notion that did not figure prominently in medical thought until the Golden Age of Greece.

Notes

1. Ebell, B. *The Papyrus Ebers.* Copenhagen: Levin and Munksgaard, 1937, p. 70.
2. Breasted, J. H. *The Edwin Smith Surgical Papyrus.* Chicago: University of Chicago Press, 1930, p. 304.

Bibliographic Commentary

In the earlier period, a few medical historians dealt with conceptual aspects of disease as supernatural. Outstanding among these were H. Sigerist, *A History of Medicine,* New York: Oxford University Press, 1951, vol. 1, and E. H. Ackerknecht, who had a series of papers in the *Bull. Hist. Med.,* "Problems of Primitive Medicine," 11:503-521, 1942; "Primitive Medicine and Culture Pattern," 12:545-574, 1942; "Psychopathology, Primitive Medicine and Primitive Culture," 14:30-67, 1943; "Natural Diseases and Rational Treatment in Primitive Medicine," 19:467-497, 1946; and "Contradictions of Primitive Surgery," 20:184-187, 1946. By the same author, see also "Natural Diseases and Rational Treatment in Primitive Medicine," *Am. Anthropologist* 47:427-432, 1945; "Primitive Medicine," *Tr. N.Y. Acad. Sci.* 8:26-37, 1946; and his essay in H. H. Walser and H. M. Koebling, eds., *Medicine and Ethnology,* Baltimore: Johns Hopkins University Press, 1971.

Nonmedical historians such as W.H.R. Rivers also evinced an early interest in primitive medicine; see his *Medicine, Magic, and Religion,* London: Kegan Paul, Trench, Trubner & Co., 1924. The subject has now become global in scope and largely the domain of anthropologists. Early classics in this regard were F. E. Clements, "Primitive Concepts of Disease," *Univ. Calif. Publications in Am. Archaeology and Ethnology* 32:185-252, 1932, the idealized structure of which was largely followed in my discussion, and the 1937 work by E. E. Evans-Pritchard, *Witchcraft, Oracles, and Magic Among the Azande,* reprinted in paperback in 1976 by Clarendon Press, London. A recent and remarkably concise overview which emphasizes sound achievements as well as theory is provided in G. P. Murdock, *Theories of Illness: A World Survey*, Pittsburgh: University of Pittsburgh Press, 1980. See also G. M. Foster and B. G. Anderson, especially the chapter "Medical Systems," in *Medical Anthropology*, New York: Wiley, 1978. A broadly based collection of essays by D. Landy, *Culture, Disease, and Healing*, New York: Macmillan, 1977, contains a section on "Medical Systems and Theories of Disease and Healing."

For a general treatment of paleopathology, see R. L. Moodie, *Paleopathology*, Urbana, Ill.: University of Illinois Press, 1923; A. T. Sandison, *Diseases in Antiquity*, Springfield, Ill.: Charles C. Thomas, 1967; S. Jarcho, ed., *Human Paleopathology*, New Haven: Yale University Press, 1966; and the section on paleopathology in Landy (see above).

The discussion of fractures in apes derives from A. H. Schutz, "Notes on Diseases and Healed Fractures of Wild Apes and Their Bearing on the Antiquity of Pathological Conditions in Man," *Bull. Hist. Med.* 7:571–582, 1939. For a summary of diseases in mummies, see A. Cockburn and E. Cockburn, *Mummies, Disease, and Ancient Cultures*, Cambridge: Cambridge University Press, 1980. An assessment of the therapeutic potential of selected ancient remedies has been provided in his fine book by G. Majno, *The Healing Hand*, Cambridge: Harvard University Press, 1975. For pitfalls in interpretation of trephination, see articles by T. D. Stewart, "Cranial Dysraphism Mistaken for Trephination," *Am. J. Phys. Anthropol.* 42:435–437, 1975, and "Are Supra-Inion Depressions Evidence of Prophylactic Trephination?" *Bull. Hist. Med.* 50:414–434, 1976. The paucity of religious emphasis by medical writers from antiquity on has been demonstrated by P. H. Kocher, "The Idea of God in Elizabethan Medicine," *J. Hist. Ideas* 11:3–29, 1950.

The role of faith in healing generally, and the Lourdes phenomenon in particular, have been studied by J. D. Frank, *Persuasion and Healing*, New York: Schocken Books, 1973, and R. H. Major, *Faiths That Healed*, New York: D. Appleton-Century Company, 1940. My account of Mary Baker Eddy derives from S. E. Ahlstrom, *A Religious History of the American People*, New Haven: Yale University Press, 1972; G. Pickering, *Creative Malady*, New York: Oxford University Press, 1974; and D. Meyer, *The Positive Thinkers*, New York: Pantheon Books, 1965. The founder gives her own version of the origins of Christian Science in M.B.G. Eddy, *Science and Health: With Keys to the Scriptures*, Boston: Joseph Armstrong, C.S.D., 1899.

A useful collection of essays on primitive thought and what might be termed psychopathology is found in A. Kiev, *Magic, Faith & Healing*, New York: Free Press, 1964.

4
DISEASE AS NATURAL AND GENERALIZED

Sooner or later, every serious reader encounters the phenomenon of the ancient Greeks. The meeting often engenders awe and, ultimately, incomprehension. The beginner should be reassured at this point that centuries of scholarship have not completely explained the epoch. In a region of the world that was already highly civilized, the Greeks emerged as a people with a revolutionary idea of the purpose of human existence and the power of the human mind.

In the process of showing what the human mind could do, the ancient Greeks placed disease on a far more rational basis than it had been before. Their accomplishment is all the more impressive because they managed it with nothing more than the same intellectual tools that had been available to all the great cultures before them – observation and rationalization. No technological advances were involved, only a remarkable extrapolation of the powers of looking and understanding. With this and little more they compiled a body of information concerning disease and its management which would be supplemented only modestly during the next thousand years.

When a modern physician is confronted with a diagnostic problem, he has all manner of technological probes at his disposal. Scarcely any nook of the human body is beyond his senses of hearing and sight. If the complaint is persistent headache, computer-assisted X rays can visualize almost any area within the skull without the necessity of surgical intervention. Delicate chemical determinations can reveal disturbed function in the pituitary or hypothalamus, structures buried in inaccessibility within the brain. Our modern physician still relies heavily on the patient's story, and he may even palpate the skull, but the final delineation of the nature of the headache will often rely on technologic resources not available to physicians prior to the mid-nineteenth century. The Greek physician, for his part, could only look and reason. Certain of them did so with surpassing skill, and the fruits of their efforts still astound the modern physician who bothers to learn about them. Greek medical writers contributed not only to their primary field of endeavor, but to the scientific scene generally. In contrast to the more important philosophers, such as Plato and Aristotle, some of the medical writers argued for the superiority of practical over theoretical knowledge. In the process they contended as well for the view that observation could be as important as rationalization, or more so. It was this belief that produced the remarkable case descriptions to which we shall return momentarily.

In early Greek medicine the name of Hippocrates has come down to us as most important. For a man so honored through the ages, surprisingly little is known of him. His birth is usually given as 460 B.C. on Cos, a small island in the eastern Aegean sea. From certain of Plato's dialogues we learn that Hippocrates was small in stature, that he was famous as a physician and teacher of physicians, and that he belonged to a healing guild called the Asklepiads. The date of his death is variously given between 380 and 370 B.C.

If this is all we know with certainty about Hippocrates, it is fair to ask, why all the bother? The answer is that for our purposes Hippocrates is important not because of the man, but because of the collection of writings that have come down in his name, some seventy books known as the *Hippocratic Corpus.* From their content it is clear that the books were not all written by Hippocrates. Indeed, it is impossible to tell which, if any, he actually authored. But little matter. We are more interested here in certain elements of thought and practice reflected by the corpus than by details of authorship.

As indicated earlier, a chief deficiency of the notion that disease is supernatural is that it ignores the ill as a source of understanding. For our purposes, the outstanding conceptual contribution in the Hippocratic writings is the notion that disease is natural. It is not known whether the Hippocratics decided a priori that disease was natural, and thus patients should be studied in the quest for understanding, or whether they fixed on disease-as-natural from some intuitive drive to observe sickness closely and at first hand. The latter would seem more reasonable, but in the Greek milieu of philosophical pursuits, the former is not inconceivable. In either event it is simply impossible to overestimate this leap in medical thinking. Without this first step scientific medicine could never have begun. If disease is natural it can be studied; it is merely one more phenomenon to be understood by observation and rationalization. And with understanding comes the possibility, at least, of control. Before considering this conceptual contribution, it should be emphasized in passing that those writers who came together under the rubric of Hippocrates did not separate themselves entirely from their origins. Elements of philosophy, certainly, and even magic and superstition can be discovered in the *Hippocratic Corpus.* Conceptual purity was no more a part of medicine in ancient Greece than it is in our own time.

To establish the Greek perception of disease as natural, we return to epilepsy, which was used earlier as an example of a malady the awesome nature of which practically invites supernatural speculation. In attacking the popular treatment of what was called the sacred disease, the Hippocratic author wrote, "For the sufferers from the disease they purify with blood and such like, as though they were polluted, bloodguilty, bewitched by men, or had committed some unholy act." He goes on to add an opposing view. "However, I hold that a man's body is not defiled by a god, the one being utterly corrupt the other perfectly holy. Nay, even should it have been defiled or in any way injured through some different agency, a god is more likely to purify and sanctify it than he is to cause defilement."[1]

Or even more explicitly, in the work entitled *On the Sacred Disease*, "It is thus with regard to the disease called Sacred: it appears to me to be nowise more divine nor sacred than other diseases, but has a natural cause from which it originates like other affections."[2]

The author goes on to give his own detailed explication of the cause of the sacred disease. In his view, the air which must move constantly throughout the body to preserve consciousness is obstructed by phlegm in the sacred disease. This explanation, erroneous in current understanding, was nonetheless natural in terms of causation. In his speculations concerning the pathology of the sacred disease, the Hippocratic writer exhibited another characteristic of the period in general. Those who criticized their contemporaries for resorting to philosophy rather than empirical observations often resorted to the same expedient, even when observation and experimentation were open to them.

Later in this exposition the writer concludes, "there is no need to put the disease in a special class and to consider it more divine than the others; they are all divine and all human." Thus he perceives all of nature as divine, and here he again falls back on philosophy, in this instance as opposed to popular religion, which would not have contended that all diseases were equally divine.[3]

Because disease as natural is seen retrospectively to be of great significance, it becomes important to demonstrate that the concept recurs in Hippocratic thinking. In *Airs, Waters, and Places,* the author speaks of the many eunuchs among the Scythians, and how popular belief holds their impotence to be a godly affliction, then concludes by saying, "but to me it appears that such affections are just as much divine as all others are, and that no one disease is either more divine or more human than another, but that all are alike divine, for that each has its own nature, and that no one arises without a natural cause."[4]

As indicated, it was the process of viewing disease as natural that led the Hippocratics to the bedside study of disease. The detailed case histories that resulted would not reappear in medical practice for over a millennium and a half. Many appear to be studies of persons suffering septicemia (blood poisoning) of a nonidentifiable type. Others are so accurately executed that, with a reasonable feeling of comfort, they can be assigned modern diagnostic terms such as malaria, puerperal (childbed) fever, and mumps. One example of their meticulous attention to detail is the description of the features of a dying person, the so-called Hippocratic facies: *"A sharp nose, hollow eyes, collapsed temples; the ears cold, contracted, and their lobes turned out; the skin about the forehead being rough, distended, and parched; the color of the whole face being green, black, livid, or lead-colored."* [5]

The *Aphorisms* produced by Hippocratic writers are masterful cameos of clinical observation. An aphorism as employed here is a short statement designed to serve as a rule of thumb for practicing physicians. Those quoted below are selected because they remain relative truisms in terms of current medical thought. It should be emphasized that many of the others would no longer be held valid by a modern clinician, if indeed he could understand them at all.

"Persons who have had frequent and severe attacks of swooning, without any manifest cause die suddenly." There is a medical condition known as the Stokes-Adams syndrome in which the heart rate is fixed at about forty beats per minute; that is, it is beating too slowly and cannot accelerate to meet ordinary demands such as exercise. Persons with this condition (now correctable by a cardiac pacemaker) frequently faint because of insufficient cerebral blood flow, and they often die suddenly from further disruption of the rhythm of the heart.

"When sleep puts an end to delirium, it is a good symptom." The delirium encountered in the Hippocratic case reports often was undoubtedly related to excessively high fevers. When such fevers suddenly break, sleep does supervene, and to that extent the observation is a sound one.

"Persons who are naturally very fat are apt to die earlier than those who are slender." This some 2,500 years before the New York Metropolitan Life Insurance Company, for actuarial purposes, compiled statistics that vindicated the Hippocratic writer.

And finally, "In acute diseases it is not quite safe to prognosticate either death or recovery," [6] a truism that young physicians today still learn happily through intuition or to their sorrow through experience. For our purposes it is not important whether a given aphorism has current application. Rather, the

significance of the aphorisms lies in their totality. Such generalizations could never have been derived by any means other than
repeated close clinical observations of illness through time, and
with some way of passing this experience on to succeeding generations of physicians. One case can produce a theory of disease,
but many are required to crystallize an aphorism.

Aphorisms were particularly adapted to the process of prognosis, which was supremely important to Greek medicine at the
time. For the most part physicians were itinerants, moving from
town to town. Reputations had to be established quickly, and for
that purpose, prognosis was more useful than therapy. Predict-
ing the outcome of a given episode of illness, and filling in symptoms forgotten by the patient, was more readily possible than
effecting a cure, which was slow if successful and uncertain in
any event.

Among those who are wont to argue such matters, the question
arises: is what the Hippocratic physicians were doing at the bedside to be dignified by the term science? In the end, as is so often
the case, the position adopted becomes a matter of semantics, a
matter of what is meant by science. For much of human history
science has been nothing more than careful observations, repeated many times so that a given phenomenon could be identified, or classified, or understood in a way that allowed prediction of its natural course. By this definition, clearly the Greek
bedside physicians were engaging in scientific activity. If, on the
other hand, the definition of science demands a prospective
experiment in which all variables are either controlled or accounted for, and can produce a statistical value of p less than
0.01, then this is not what the Hippocratics were doing. But neither does the latter definition describe much modern clinical research, although the individuals so engaged today would take
considerable umbrage at the suggestion that they were not
scientific.

Certain it is that at least some Hippocratic writers understood
the problem and believed they were acting scientifically. In the
Precepts we read, "One must attend in medical practice not primarily to plausible theories, but to experience combined with
reason. . . . Now I approve of theorising also if it lays its founda-

tion in incident (facts), and deduces its conclusions in accordance with phenomena."[7]

On the other hand the case for Hippocratic physicians as scientists can easily be overstated. More recent scholarship has established at least one fact: the matter is not as black and white as it is set up to be by some observers. Quite apart from the position one arrives at in this debate, the accomplishments of Greek physicians during this time stand on their merits regardless of any discussion of the nature of science.

Professionalization

With the Greeks medicine began on the road to professionalization. One measure of this is the Hippocratic Oath (see the appendix), the earliest known attempt of a group to police itself internally, which is one stamp of a profession.

The origin of the oath appears to have been Pythagorean rather than Hippocratic, but more recent scholarship suggests that some of what was interpreted earlier as Pythagorean may have reflected popular ethical influences instead. In either event it was not until early Christian times that the oath was accepted or even noticed by medical writers in Greece or Rome. Putting aside the question of the oath's origin and the matter of its delayed adoption, the fact that it was taken up by any school of medicine indicates a striving for professionalization.

Disease as Generalized in Origin

The oath is mentioned in passing because it ties in with the second major aspect of the Greek conception of disease, which is that disease is generalized in its origin. It is likely that Greek medicine was practiced on at least two levels, that of the leech and that of the physician. The principal distinction between the two was that for the leech medicine was a craft, for the physician, a science. Laying aside the details, we will be interested principally in the fact that the physician, as a scientist, had to underpin his profession with theory. In part that was because physicians could expect to encounter strange new illnesses wherein theory alone and not experience could provide the requisite flexibility.

It was a return to the theorizing of philosophy that led the Hippocratics to conclude that disease resulted from a generalized imbalance of the fluid portion of the body. Herein they departed from the bedside observations that had produced the idea of disease as natural. One aspect of Greek philosophy at this juncture was the search for uniformity in the otherwise bewildering complexity of natural phenomena. As far back as the pre-Socratics, Greek philosophers had struggled after uniformity in the elemental makeup of the world. Earlier the Babylonians, then the Egyptians, had supposed that first water, then air and earth were the primary constituents of the world. Variously, pre-Socratic Greek philosophers adopted one or the other of these and added a fourth, fire. Empedocles, a contemporary of Hippocrates, carried the theory a bit further when he proposed that all mortal things were made up of varying proportions of these four elements. In their quest for the elemental substance these philosophers were not concerned with the problems facing physicians, who were searching for an understanding of the mechanisms of disease. As we have seen, however, given the general role of philosophy in Greek thought at the time, it is not surprising that physicians would adapt philosophical constructs to their medical theorization.

The four elements—earth, water, fire, and air—were characterized by specific qualities. Earth was dry and cold; fire, dry and hot; air, hot and wet; water, wet and cold. The human body, or more specifically its fluid portion, was composed of four principal humors—blood, phlegm, yellow bile, and black bile. These humors were characterized by the same four qualities, so that black bile was dry and cold; yellow bile, dry and hot; blood, hot and wet; phlegm, wet and cold.

To all this the Hippocratics added the notion of balance or harmony, and the theory was then related to disease as follows: "The body of man has in itself blood, phlegm, yellow bile and black bile; these make up the nature of his body, and through these he feels pain or enjoys health. Now he enjoys the most perfect health when these elements are duly proportioned to one another in respect of compounding, power and bulk, and when they are perfectly mingled."[8] Diagnosis, then, was a matter of recognizing which of the humors was imbalanced and to what extent, and treatment was directed at reestablishing equilibrium.

In admittedly simplified form, the system worked as follows. If the patient presented a common cold, clearly there was an excess of phlegm. The qualities of phlegm are wet and cold. The opposite of phlegm is yellow bile, whose qualities are hot and dry. Treatment must either diminish phlegm or enhance yellow bile. The patient might be advised to go to bed and to drink moderate amounts of wine, thus increasing dryness and heat. Where this particular malady is concerned, treatment has changed in 2,500 years only by the substitution of whiskey for wine, an innovation of dubious value.

Using a purely philosophical foundation, then, the Greeks arrived at a modus operandi for disease that is almost precisely opposed to our own. For the Greeks disease arose in a general imbalance in the fluid portion of the body, although it could produce localized symptoms. In this system fever might result from an excess of blood, but there is no reason that this morbid condition might not manifest itself as a yellow skin and swollen spleen. In current theory disease arises locally in the solid portion of the body (cells or subcellular structures) and may have either localized or generalized manifestations. Thus hyperthyroidism, caused by the local overproduction of thyroid hormone, may present clinically with a rapid pulse, hot skin, nervousness, tremor, weight loss, and weakness, none of which appears directly related to the localized swelling in the neck that is responsible for the symptoms.

Thyroid disease and similar endocrine disorders are seized upon occasionally by casual students of history as exoneration of the basic Hippocratic notion of disease as imbalance. Endocrine disease results when there is too much (hyperthyroidism) or too little (hypothyroidism) hormone, and greatest health prevails when there is precisely enough (euthyroidism). The leap from Hippocratic balance to euthyroidism is of course too great. The concept of disease as too much or too little, as we have seen, is common in primitive constructs as well. The difference lies in understanding what it is there is too little or too much of, and yellow bile is not thyroxine. Many medical innovators have been right for the wrong reasons in the history of humankind. Indeed, at times actions taken for the wrong reasons have turned out to be beneficial, but even then they should not be accorded any distinction beyond that which is duly theirs, and so it must be with the Hippocratics and the conception of disease as imbalance.

The Hippocratics transcended the other ancient schools of medical thought because of their ethical ideals that contributed to professionalization, because of their heavy influence on Western medicine as it later developed, and because of their emphasis on the careful study of individual illnesses, which grew out of the concept of disease as natural.

It now becomes possible to take two leaps in time, one of 500 years, the other of 1,000 years. Such telescoping would be out of the question if we were considering the history of medicine rather than concepts of disease. The Hippocratics envisioned disease as natural in origin and mediated by a generalized imbalance in the fluid portion of the body, notably the four humors. In the ensuing centuries as Greek thought spread around the Mediterranean, differing schools of thought arose. These sects came into being not because of innovations in diagnosis or treatment, but because of philosophical differences in their conception of disease causation.

One such school of thought, the Empiricists, eschewed all theorization and experimentation, preferring to rely on experience alone. Thus they paid no attention to causation beyond such obvious factors as inadequate nutrition and climatic conditions. A second, the Methodists, dates from the first century B.C., and as their name implies, they reduced disease and its treatment to an easily manageable scheme. Disease was characterized by *status laxus,* an excessive relaxation of the body's internal pores; *status strictus,* the opposite situation; or *status mixtus,* whose meaning is obvious. Treatment was directed at relaxing the excessively narrow and narrowing the excessively relaxed.

The Empiricists and the Methodists enjoyed a wide vogue in their time, but both had faded by the time we return to the Hippocratic thread in Rome in the second century A.D. Here we encounter a Greek physician, Galen, who with a number of compatriots had by this time established Greek thought and practice as the dominant force in Roman medicine.

Galen was born about A.D. 130 and died about 200. The son of an architect in Pergamon in Asia Minor, he studied medicine abroad for nine years before returning home to become surgeon to the gladiators. Later he journeyed to Rome, where after a time he became a famous physician. Though he frequently alluded to Hippocrates in reverent terms and managed to associate his name with the father of medicine throughout the Middle Ages, Galen was more than a mere follower of Hippocrates. Where the Hippocratics had cared little for the basic medical sciences, Galen was a first-rate anatomist and physiologist. His biological experiments far surpassed any that had been executed before him or would be for more than a thousand years thereafter. But this is another story, to which we return in considering the concept of experimental medicine.

Our present interest in Galen relates to his pathology, which was humoral. He took the doctrine of the four humors, elaborated and polished it, and wrote about it so extensively and authoritatively that it remained the reigning theory of disease causation for some 1,500 years. Because of this influence Galen is often reviled as a negative influence on the development of medicine. Such a charge is akin to blaming Christ for the Inquisition. The fact is that Galenic pathology prevailed in the West because no greater medical mind appeared during the Middle Ages, because of the conservatism and authoritarianism that characterized the period, because he left a theory that united the available medical science, and because he saw the human body in teleological terms; that is, he considered human structures to be perfectly designed for their assigned functions – a doctrine that rendered Galen acceptable to Roman Catholicism as it came to control the intellectual life of the Latin West.

At this point our conceptual byway comes to a fork, and neither road need occupy us at length. With the decline of Rome, Greek medical thought atrophied in the Latin West. The little that survived was preserved between roughly A.D. 500 and 1000 in the monasteries that became the only significant repositories of knowledge. From A.D. 1000 to 1200 or so, a lay school developed at Salerno, leavened by new translations of ancient Greek works, after which the medieval universities dominated the scene and an imperfect Galenism ruled medical teaching and practice.

By then the Eastern branch of Greek thought was traversing

North Africa and centering in Spain. This came about through the dynamic spread of Islamic thought beginning in the seventh century A.D. Greek medicine at the time was centered in Gundeshapur, where it had been carried by a Christian sect, the Nestorians, who had been driven from the Byzantine realm for religious reasons. From Gundeshapur, ancient medical thought was transmitted to Syrians and Arabs, the latter carrying it finally to their Western caliphate in Spain. To cities such as Cordoba, beginning in the eleventh century, scholars from all over Europe flocked to complete the circle of translations back to Latin from the Arabic.

By this torturous route, then, disease as natural and generalized, dressed in the garb of humoral pathology, rose to ascendancy in the minds of our own medical progenitors. To be sure it was not identical with Galen's version of the four humors, but the elements were there. At various times more or less emphasis was put on the four temperaments, that is, the human constitution as modified by the individual's dominance by phlegmatic, choleric, sanguine, or melancholy influences, a notion with roots that go back to Hippocratic times. The system was further modified by astrological thinking, an influence that would not diminish until the Renaissance. In its application, the system was so complex and alien to later medical thinking that a modern physician can scarcely make sense of it.

The conception of disease as natural was a beneficent contribution because it encouraged the study of disease and the possibility of human intervention in the process of illness. In short, it enhanced clinical or bedside medicine. The other half of the Hippocratic-Galenic legacy, the notion that disease originates as an imbalance in the generalized fluid portion of the body, had a stultifying effect on what we now term the basic sciences of medicine – anatomy, physiology, biochemistry, pathology. We will see that Galen himself believed strongly in the value of dissection and experimentation. Yet in truth there is little need for anatomical knowledge in a system of humoral pathology. Diagnosis and treatment do not depend on a full and detailed knowledge of the body's anatomical arrangements. So it was that as long as humoral pathology dominated medical thinking, little research was likely to develop. In Galen's writings, embellished by Arabic additions, all that needed to be known was known.

We have seen how one conception of disease held sway over Western medical thought throughout most of the Christian era. In the next segment of the story we will find that a few individuals began to depart from certain aspects of Galenic teachings as early as the sixteenth century. But, in general, humoral pathology, with variations on the theme, continued as the mainstream of medical thinking down to the nineteenth century. Vesalius was to revolutionize Galenic anatomy; Harvey would disprove the Galenic notion of the movement of the blood; Sydenham would conclude that there were specific diseases; but none of these illustrious innovators would be able to remove himself entirely from humoral thinking. It was not until physicians became heavily imbued with anatomical thinking and received improved tools of physical diagnosis that the origin of disease as localized would become the medical mode. That story can begin with the amazingly fruitful construct that came to be known as the anatomical idea, a story that will take us into relatively recent times.

Notes

1. Jones, H.W.S. *Hippocrates.* London: William Heinemann, 1923, vol. 2, p. 149.
2. Adams, F. *The Genuine Works of Hippocrates.* New York: William Wood and Company, 1886, vol. 2, p. 334.
3. Lloyd, G.E.R. "Aspects of the Interrelationships of Medicine, Magic and Philosophy in Ancient Greece," *Apeiron* 9:5, 1975.
4. Adams, *Genuine Works of Hippocrates.* Vol. 1, p. 178.
5. Ibid., p. 195.
6. The four aphorisms are from Adams, vol. 2, pp. 208, 200, 209, and 204 respectively.
7. Jones, *Hippocrates.* Vol. 1, p. 313.
8. Ibid., vol. 4, p. 11.

Bibliographic Commentary

The principal earlier translations of Hippocratic writings are the ten volumes of E. Littré, *Oeuvres Complètes d'Hippocrate,* Paris: J. B. Baillière, 1839–1861; the uncompleted work of I. Ilberg and H. Kuehlewein, *Hippocratis Opera Quae Feruntur Omnia,* Leipzig: B. G. Teubner, 1894–1902; W.H.S. Jones, *Hippocrates,* London: W. Heinemann, 1923–1931, 4 vols. (vol. 3 by E. T. Withington); and F. Adams, *The Genuine Works of Hippocrates,* New York: William Wood and Company, 1886. Later interpretations of ancient Greek medical writings include H.

Sigerist, *A History of Medicine,* vol. 2, New York: Oxford University Press, 1961; O. Temkin, "Greek Medicine as Science and Craft," reprinted in *The Double Face of Janus,* Baltimore: Johns Hopkins University Press, 1977; and the three works by G.E.R. Lloyd, *Early Greek Science: Thales to Aristotle,* London: Chatto and Windus, 1970; *Greek Science After Aristotle,* by the same publisher, 1973; and *Hippocratic Writings,* New York: Penguin Books, 1978. The most recent textbook covering Greek medicine in Rome is J. Scarborough, *Roman Medicine,* Ithaca: Cornell University Press, 1969.

The sacred disease is treated in detail in O. Temkin, *The Falling Sickness,* Baltimore: Johns Hopkins University Press, rev. ed., 1971, and G.E.R. Lloyd, "Aspects of the Interrelationships of Medicine, Magic and Philosophy in Ancient Greece," *Apeiron* 9:1-16, 1975.

The seminal treatment of the Hippocratic Oath is L. Edelstein, *The Hippocratic Oath,* supp. no. 1 to *Bull. Hist. Med.,* Baltimore: Johns Hopkins University Press, 1943. For a partial revision of Edelstein's revisionist theory, see F. Kudlien, "Medical Ethics and Popular Ethics in Greece and Rome," *Clio Medica* 5:91-121, 1970. Galen's medical philosophy is treated specifically by O. Temkin, *Galenism,* Ithaca: Cornell University Press, 1973. G.E.R. Lloyd analyzes the qualities of the humors in "The Hot and the Cold, the Dry and the Wet in Greek Philosophy," *J. Hellenistic Studies* 84:92-106, 1964.

5
THE ANATOMICAL
IDEA

The year 1500 is often encountered as marking the beginning of the modern era. Historians recognize the artificiality of such designations but continue to use them for the sake of convenience. If it is to be viewed broadly, a form as complex as human history requires some sort of skeletal landmarks. The inadequacies of sharply drawn epochal designations are likewise widely known. The medieval period is often portrayed as intellectually sterile, but an era that gave us Petrarch, Dante, Chaucer, and Boccaccio in secular literature and Aquinas in theology cannot be characterized so easily. The Middle Ages also produced the beginnings of four great institutions of medicine – universities, hospitals, public health, and nursing as a profession. It is true that the major medieval contributions came in later centuries, but at no time does one find the near total darkness some formerly associated with the period.

Yet it is also true that if one examines the institutions and ideas of Western Europe in the sixteenth and seventeenth centuries, one readily concludes that profound changes had occurred. Human life was no longer a mere preparation for a better life hereafter, but a time for exercising mature freedom as a part of nature and even for enjoying the earthly stay, an outlook that derived from a return to the literature of the classical periods of Greece and Rome. And further, our idealized sixteenth- and seventeenth-century man gradually had divested himself of the notion that there was only the truth of Christianity, whether Roman Catholic or Protestant. Rather, he was coming to believe that there existed as yet unrevealed truth that could be discovered by human effort, even if only slowly and with difficulty. This latter was the revival of rationalism, and its method was that of science.

No one can point to a year as the beginning of Protestantism, humanism, or rationalism, because all of these ideas had pre-Renaissance origins. Protestantism did not really begin in 1517, when Luther posted his ninety-five theses on Wittenberg Church; nor did humanism come to life only after 1494, when Pico's *Oration* was posthumously published, revealing his doctrine of the dignity of man; nor did rationalism begin in 1605, when Francis Bacon published the *Advancement of Learning*, spelling out many of the aspects of the new science, which would be developed more fully fifteen years later in his *Novum Organum*. Several generations of scholars and scientists can be identified in which ideas and practices coexisted that we might now label as characteristically medieval or Renaissance in nature. In the history of disease perhaps no one better exemplifies this transitional period than Paracelsus, who lived from 1493 or 1494 to 1541.

There is an element of irony in introducing the development of anatomical thinking with the elusive Paracelsus, as he has been called, considering the fact that he had essentially no use for anatomy as the discipline is now employed. For our purposes Paracelsus is useful for quite a different reason, which should become apparent as we go along. He was born of German-Swiss stock and given a name which in a later Latinized form became Philippus Aureolus Theophrastus Bombastus von Hohenheim. His nature proved as formidable as his name, both to his contemporaries and to later historians.

Paracelsus is often lionized as the first significant medical man to make a telling break with Galen. With this there can be no general dispute, and indeed, this is my main reason for recruiting him at this point. He specifically rejected Galen and Hippocrates as the source of his medical knowledge and relied instead on first-hand experience. From this, with characteristic vehemence, he denied the doctrine of the four humors as the cause of all disease. Perhaps to dramatize his rejection of ancient authority, he lectured and wrote in the German vernacular, an unheard-of departure which contributed to the rejection by both colleagues and students that was finally his fate. Indisputably, here was more than a zephyr of fresh air.

But Paracelsus cannot be judged merely by his rebelliousness. His place in history would be far less elusive if he had left a more utilitarian edifice in place of the one he tried, but failed, to destroy. But instead of the discarded four humors, he explained health and disease within a system of five spheres, the whole of which was ultimately as speculative as the doctrine of the four humors. Instead of air, fire, water, and earth, for Paracelsus all bodies were made up of the three chemical principles, mercury, sulfur, and salt. His abandonment of traditional polypharmacy in favor of metallic therapy was one of Paracelsus's larger contributions, but this was progress only if the new chemicals were genuinely efficacious, or at least less dangerous than the traditional drugs, an arguable conclusion to say the least. He retained a heavy emphasis on uroscopy (diagnosis by inspecting the urine), which is difficult to square with his emphasis on experience as the only valid instructor, and he could not bring himself to discard astrology.

When all the confusing trappings are stripped away, insofar as they can be, Paracelsus's scientific method is seen to be "intuitive and interpretative." He insists that the only worthwhile book is the book of nature, but he provides no method for its use. The book is there, but it is up to each individual to do his own reading. Small wonder that he left no effective disciples to further the break with tradition that he strove so mightily to launch.

Yet, while the controversial Swiss left no immediate school of followers, some thirty years later there had developed a Paracelsian school of physicians, which featured a new outlook that called for the renunciation of tradition for its own sake and summoned up a new medicine based on personal observations. Herein lies Paracelsus's significance for our story. It is not that he directly improved mankind's ability to control disease, but rather he is seen as a Janus of sorts, one face directed backwards to his medieval heritage, the other looking forward to the changes he desired but could not effect. He demonstrates that humanism and rationalism, the forces for change that were already at work in religious reformation, were poised to move medical men as well. The most significant early effect of the new *Zeitgeist* was to be a scientific and accurate human anatomy that provided Renaissance man an entirely new view of his microcosm, and Paracelsus tells us that the time for that was now ripe.

Early Anatomical Study

There was little hope for a scientific anatomy until dissection of the human body could be made more acceptable, a climate that resulted from the same basic forces that forged Renaissance changes generally. For a variety of reasons many societies have abhorred and even proscribed the dissection of the recently dead. The opposing idea, which held that the body became insignificant after death, began to appear as early as ancient Greece, particularly in the mind of Socrates as reflected in the writings of Plato.

After Alexandria's founding in the fourth century B.C. and its ascendancy to the role of "the acropolis of classical knowledge," the scientific approach to anatomy was carried to heights that would not be seen in Western Europe until the sixteenth century. The two principals here were Herophilus (born in the late fourth century B.C.) and Erasistratus (born ca. 304 B.C.), whose many contributions to basic medical science, none of which has come down to us in complete form, need not concern us here. What they signify to us is that human dissection became relatively commonplace during this era. Indeed, if we are to believe the account of the Roman medical writer Celsus (first century A.D.), Herophilus and Erasistratus went even further, to engage in vivisections on prisoners supplied by the kings.

The great surge in anatomical investigation in Alexandria had diminished by 150 B.C., and under Roman dominion dissection became difficult once more. Largely because the available source material is so scarce, historians currently dispute the importance of Alexandria in later centuries. The best estimate is that with peaks and valleys the center remained a magnet for students and a focus of excellent medical teaching into the fourth century A.D.

Much of what we know of Herophilus and Erasistratus was recorded by Galen (born 129 or 130, died 199 or 200 A.D.), who himself represented the high-water mark in anatomical thinking between the golden era of Alexandrian biology and the Renaissance. As we have seen, much of his physiology and pathology drew upon traditional ideas, but in anatomical investigation, Galen was truly innovative. He recognized that ideally dissection should be on human bodies, but it is certain that he rarely had such opportunity and possible that all his dissections were limited to animals. His motives for studying anatomy included immediate application of the knowledge thus derived for purposes of surgical practice. His enforced reliance on animal dissection led Galen to numerous errors when he extrapolated his findings to human beings, but these should be weighed against his very real achievements. He insisted on first-hand experience in dissection, resorted to vivisection where it was indicated, and in the process compiled the anatomical authority which would dominate the field for centuries.

Pre-Vesalian Anatomy

Although dissection continued in the Byzantine Empire, it was bound to diminish in the Arabic sphere of influence and remained uncommon in the Latin West up to the waning of the Middle Ages. It appears that the papacy never directly prohibited human dissection. This leaves a problem in explaining why a number of medieval physicians saw it as a sin. At one point the pre-Vesalian anatomist Mondino (ca. 1275–1326) observed that the bones of the skull were better seen if boiled, but hastened to add that he eschewed the process because of the sin involved. Mondino's statement gives a clue to one reason dissection may have been viewed as sin in the absence of any formal papal pronouncement. During the centuries before Mondino, a practice had developed of boiling the bones of persons who died in distant lands so that their remains might be interred in home ground. This became so popular during the Crusades that Pope Boniface VIII in 1299 issued a bull prohibiting the practice. It is possible that this edict was misinterpreted, either inadvertently by certain well-meaning clerics or deliberately by the more zealous among them. In any event, strong societal pressures, including religion, held human dissection to a minimum until near the end of the Middle Ages.

Beginning in the fourteenth century, particularly in Italy and most especially Bologna, things began to change. For legal reasons such as suspected poisonings, and at times to try to discover the cause of disease, human dissection began to increase. Gradually it became an accepted practice in the universities, where it was an annual or biennial event, a sort of academic holiday in which all teachers and students took part, not just those of a medical persuasion. In 1340 a university statute was passed in Montpellier providing for a biennial anatomy, and Parliament extended a similar privilege to the barber-surgeons of England two centuries later, when it passed an act that handed over for dissection four individuals each year who had been executed as criminals.

So we find a more liberal climate for dissection arriving with the Renaissance. In the first half of the sixteenth century, this movement was catalyzed not through the efforts of physicians but of artists. The return to classical forms pervaded many aspects of Renaissance life, not just that of ideas. Artists, too, were caught up in the new spirit. The human being was the greatest of God's creations. What better way to glorify the Almighty than to depict His greatest work in its classical nude form? When they consulted existing medical texts it became clear to the artists that they would have to obtain their anatomical knowledge firsthand, either from observing or from taking part in dissections.

The greatest of these artist-dissectors was the awesome Renaissance figure Leonardo da Vinci (1452-1519). After dissecting perhaps as few as ten or as many as thirty different bodies, Leonardo compiled a series of anatomical drawings that were far superior to any in existing medical texts. Their excellence was marvelled at by a contemporary, and they remain a remarkable achievement even to eyes accustomed to modern anatomical illustration. Having said all this, it remains to conclude that the dissections undertaken by Renaissance artists, even the transcendental accomplishment of Leonardo, had little direct effect on the development of anatomy as a science. In part this relates to the reason Renaissance artists had for dissecting. In anatomy, as in science generally, the answers derived from an experiment usually depend on the questions asked. If one opens a human body to remove the internal organs in preparation for embalming, as the ancient Egyptians did in the process of mummification, the likelihood is great that little medically useful anatomical information will be obtained. The same outcome is probable if the purpose of the incision is to look for poison or some other cause of death. In short, a dissection is not always an anatomy.

The painters and sculptors of the sixteenth century were seeking anatomical knowledge only insofar as it served their art. They needed only the general configuration of the body, largely the skin, bony structure, and superficial muscles, what is termed topographic anatomy. They had no need to dissect out the sciatic nerve from its beginning at the fourth and fifth lumbar and first, second, and third sacral nerves to its termination in the skin of the foot. There were occasional exceptions to this statement. Leonardo's compulsive curiosity, for example, led him to dissections within the bodily cavities, but even for him this was unusual.

Further, the artists had no particular reason to bother themselves with the names of the structures they were seeing. Anatomical terminology, much of it Arabic at this time, was still confused and rudimentary, a situation which hindered the artists' efforts and which they, including Leonardo, did nothing to improve. Finally, da Vinci's drawings, which certainly could have aided physicians had they been printed and distributed, were scattered and not generally known until late in the nineteenth century.

Even though Renaissance artists were not anatomists in the scientific sense, their efforts indirectly abetted the development of scientific anatomy. Their contribution was the aid they lent the popularization of dissection. They helped produce an ambiance in which anatomical studies could be pursued by physicians for medical purposes. That opportunity was seized by a number of individuals in the fifteenth and first half of the sixteenth century, all of whom we must necessarily pass by to get to the figure whose efforts eclipsed everything that had happened in medical science in the thirteen hundred years since Galen's death.

Vesalius and the Advent of Scientific Anatomy

Andreas Vesalius was born in Brussels on New Year's night, forcing his biographers to choose between the years 1514 and

1515, and died in 1564. He studied medicine at Paris, Louvain, and his native city before succumbing to the lure of the hospitable medical climate south of the Alps, specifically Padua in Italy. There, on December 5, 1537, he took his doctor's degree, and the next day, at age twenty-three, was appointed professor of surgery and anatomy. With this event there accelerated at Padua a tradition of excellence in anatomy which would draw students from all over Europe in the years that followed.

From the beginning of his academic career, Vesalius broke with tradition in a way that appears simple at first glance, but which eventually proved crucial to his success. When he appeared on the scene of academic anatomy, the prevailing practice had the professor of anatomy uninvolved in firsthand dissection. Rather, he sat in an elevated chair (*cathedra*) at the head of the table, reading from an anatomy text. The dissection was performed by a barber or surgeon or medical student, and the anatomical landmarks mentioned by the professor were then pointed out to the assemblage by a second assistant known as an ostensor. Vesalius would have none of this. He had become an accomplished dissector as a student and, as Galen before him, had learned the pitfalls inherent in relying on assistants for dissection.

At about this time Vesalius was approached by a printer who wished the young professor to assist in the preparation of a new edition of Galen's anatomy. Now in possession of both of Galen's major anatomical works and deeply engaged in his own dissections, Vesalius was discovering one Galenic error after another. The liver did not have four or five lobes nor the sternum seven parts. The lower jaw did not consist of two parts nor was the uterus horned in shape. How had Galen arrived at such misconceptions? To Vesalius the answer was soon clear. Galen had never or rarely dissected a human body, nor had he claimed to. The assumption that he had done so was a natural error promulgated over the years by physicians who did not have access to all of Galen's writings. This revelation was important to Vesalius for at least two reasons. It gave him courage to challenge the previously unassailable Galen while simultaneously excusing the prince of physicians for the misinterpretation others had put on his work. It also convinced Vesalius more than ever that he must press on with a project he already had under way – an entirely new anatomy based on his own extensive human dissections.

Even though the popular prejudice against dissection had diminished, the problem of obtaining suitable specimens persisted. To obtain a skeleton for his own use, Vesalius had stolen the corpse of an executed criminal from the gibbet, and now as he worked on what would be his *magnum opus,* he was still forced at times to engage in grave robbing. In addition to the unprecedented accuracy of his text, Vesalius oversaw the execution of illustrations which not only gave a new dimension to anatomical illustration, but even today are regarded as works of art in their own right. For years the art work was credited to Johann Stepan von Kalkar, but this point is now debated. What is not disputed is that the results are superb examples of the fully realized potential of the woodcut in medical illustration. In what must have been an anxious time for Vesalius, the precious woodcuts were transported by mule over the Alps to the Greek scholar and printer J. Oporinus of Basle. In 1543 the book appeared as *De humani corporis fabrica libri septum* (On the Fabric of the Human Body in Seven Books), or less cumbersomely, the *Fabrica.* In the same year Copernicus brought out his main work, *De revolutionibus orbium coelestium* (On the Revolution of the Celestial Orbs), in which he placed the sun rather than the Earth at the center of the solar system. Thus, as has been observed, the year 1543 handed mankind a revolutionary new way of looking at both his microcosm and his macrocosm.

The reception of the *Fabrica* was predictable. By now Galen's authority in medical matters approximated that of the Bible in religious questions. Suddenly there had appeared a twenty-eight-year-old upstart who accused the universally accepted authority of all manner of error. In truth it was only with difficulty that Vesalius had wrenched himself free of Galen's influence. In his early years on the faculty at Padua, he had lectured three times on the bones as depicted by Galen before mustering sufficient courage to call attention to the errors. And in the *Fabrica,* when it became necessary to contradict Galen, Vesalius strove for circumspection, at least by the standards of a century that not infrequently produced exhortations of the sort associated with Benvenuto Cellini. In his scheme of motion of the blood, for example, Galen was forced to postulate pores in the septum dividing the heart in order to get blood from the right to the left side. When it came to these pores Vesalius wrote in paraphrase, "God is wonderful and Galen says the pores are there, but let's be clear on one point; I have not seen them."

Many rushed to condemn Vesalius, but none with the ferocity of his old teacher in Paris, Sylvius, who played maliciously on Vesalius's name by dubbing him *vesanus*, or madman, and who explained the errors in Galen's anatomy by concluding that the human body had changed, but not for the better. It remained for his students, as only students can, to repay Sylvius in kind. On his tomb they added an epitaph of their own.

> In this grave lies old Sylvius, during his day
> He never gave aught without getting full pay;
> And though dead as a herring, so nought could be worse,
> He is vexed he can't charge you for reading this verse.

There is no need to belabor the case for the greatness of Vesalius's contribution. It is true that the time was ready for the appearance of a scientific anatomy, and indeed another man, Giambattista Canano (1515-1579), was working along the same lines, when he probably saw the excellent illustrations from Vesalius's books and so abandoned his own work. The *Fabrica* is all the testimony Vesalius requires, and it is the book that interests us here.

The importance of anatomical thinking can be exaggerated, as we shall see in what follows, but only with difficulty. It gave rise to a construct historians have labeled the anatomical idea, a concept that came into being, matured slowly, and finally led medical men to the amazingly fruitful conclusion that disease was localized in origin. It must be emphasized again that the anatomical idea did not originate with Vesalius. The Alexandrian biologists, Galen, and the numerous pre-Vesalian anatomists of the late Middle Ages and early Renaissance have already been cited for their structural thinking. The anatomical idea, rather, is a historical device used to trace the thread of anatomical thinking in the conceptual tapestry of medical thought during the centuries after the publication of the *Fabrica*.

The anatomical idea is so simple and basic to present thinking that students have difficulty understanding why it was so long delayed in terms of influencing what physicians thought and did about disease. The concept holds that the body is composed of interrelated anatomical units and that the arrangement of these units has much to say about the way the body functions (physiology). By extension, disruption in the relationships among these units can produce localized disease (pathology), the signs and symptoms of which may also depend upon the anatomical arrangements (physical diagnosis).

The first of these steps, from the study of structure to that of function, was made contemporaneously with the beginnings of scientific anatomy. The flow of thinking from structure to function is so logical it might almost be termed natural. If handed a nondescript box and asked to determine its function, one would almost certainly open it to see if anything about its internal structure revealed its purpose. Leonardo saw as much and even went so far as to replace the muscles of the arm and leg with cords attached to the bones to demonstrate the actions of levers and pulleys. The same easy transition from structure to function was revealed by Vesalius. In the last book of the *Fabrica*, there is a section on experiments with living creatures indicating the clear separation, yet natural connection, between physiology and anatomy. Inherent kinship of structure and function will be treated at greater length when we take up the concept of experimental medicine. For the moment, we turn instead to trace the anatomical idea as it led to the concept of localized disease.

Bibliographic Commentary

Paracelsus remains, perhaps, the most enigmatic major figure in the history of medicine. His principal biography is by W. Pagel, *Paracelsus*, Basel: S. Karger, 1958. In something approaching desperation, Sigerist concluded that possibly only Germans could ever understand the mercurial Paracelsus, in *Henry E. Sigerist on the History of Medicine*, New York: MD Publications, 1960. Owsei Temkin has written a helpful essay, "The Elusiveness of Paracelsus," in *The Double Face of Janus*, Baltimore: Johns Hopkins University Press, 1977. E. H. Ackerknecht's assessment of Paracelsus is refreshingly objective, in "Recurrent Themes in Medical Thought," *Scientific Monthly* 69:80–83, 1949, and "Aspects of the History of Therapeutics," *Bull. Hist. Med.* 36:389–419, 1962. The persistence of Paracelsian influence was traced by A. Debus, *The English Paracelsians*, London: Oldbourne, 1965.

The accomplishments of the Alexandrian anatomists are assessed by G.E.R.

Lloyd, *Greek Science After Aristotle,* London: Chatto and Windus, 1973, and by P. Potter, "Herophilus of Chalcedon: An Assessment of His Place in the History of Anatomy," *Bull. Hist. Med.* 50:45-60, 1976.

The question of the enduring influence of Alexandrian science is found in J. Scarborough, "Ammianus Marcellinus XXII. 16. 18: Alexandria's Medical Reputation in the Fourth Century," *Clio Medica* 4:141-142, 1969, and in the critique by V. Nutton, "Ammianus and Alexandria," *Clio Medica* 7:165-176, 1972.

A short, highly readable account of Galen is by G. Sarton, *Galen of Pergamon,* Lawrence: University of Kansas Press, 1954. The changes undergone by Galen and his influence are traced by O. Temkin, *Galenism,* Ithaca: Cornell University Press, 1973.

Leonardo da Vinci's anatomical drawings, as well as his place in the development of anatomy, are most conveniently found in C. D. O'Malley and J. B. de C. M. Saunders, *Leonardo da Vinci on the Human Body,* New York: Henry Schuman, 1952. Anatomy before Vesalius has been exhaustively explored by L. R. Lind, *Studies in Pre-Vesalian Anatomy,* Philadelphia: American Philosophical Society, 1975. The development of attitudes toward dissection is traced in the biographical study by C. D. O'Malley, *Andreas Vesalius of Brussels, 1514-1564,* Berkeley: University of California Press, 1965. A critical study of the illustrations in the *Fabrica* is J. B. de C. M. Saunders and C. D. O'Malley, *The Illustrations from the Works of Andreas Vesalius of Brussels,* Cleveland: World Publishing Company, 1950.

6
DISEASE AS LOCALIZED

Localization in Antiquity

Although the notion that disease originates locally did not dominate medical thinking in any practical way until the nineteenth century, it should not surprise us that the roots of the idea can be traced much further back. In antiquity Aretaeus appears to have known that injury to one side of the brain paralyzes the opposite side of the body, and there is definite evidence of localized thinking in the Hippocratic writings, for example in the aphorisms. Also in these writings is a group which has come to be known as the Cnidian treatises, and they are of particular interest to the concept at hand. Traditionally it has been believed that two major schools of medical thought existed in the Aegean region during the fifth and fourth centuries B.C. The Hippocratic school centered on the island of Cos, as we have seen, conceived disease largely as generalized in its origin and manifestations. Cnidus, a city situated thirty miles to the east, featured a school in which localization of disease was an important consideration. Recent scholarship debates the question of whether the two schools were distinct and competitive during the period in question or whether the idea of two contending schools was made up by scholars influenced by the fact that distinctly separate medical sects did exist later during the Hellenistic period.

Certainly there is valid disagreement over which of the Hippocratic writings should be labeled as Cnidian, but the finer points
of this complex issue need not subvert our present purpose.
Whether or not they derived from a distinct and competitive
school at the time, the treatises now identified as Cnidian indicate distinct localized thinking as far back as the Golden Age of
Greece. In the Cnidian system, bile and phlegm were inborn and
permanent ingredients of the body. Disease could be produced
by a combination of internal and external causes, but the final
common pathway, the pathologic lesion, consisted of localized
deposits of bile and phlegm which had become coagulated. From
this reasoning came a system of disease which, in part, featured
seven diseases caused by bile, twelve of the bladder, four of the
kidneys, three types of tetanus, four stranguries (difficulty in
evacuating the urine), four forms of icterus (jaundice), and three
of phthisis. Although mixed with what we would now term
symptoms (icterus, strangury), the Cnidian system also clearly
featured localization at the organ level (bladder, kidneys).

Erasistratus, whom we encountered because of his anatomical
achievements in Alexandria in the middle of the third century
B.C., abandoned humoral pathology in favor of an anatomical approach to disease. In truth, he went far down the ontological
road, writing on such diseases as paralysis, dropsy, and gout. But
his lead was not followed by those who came after him. Galen,
whom I earlier credited with polishing the notion of disease as
generalized, when the complete record is consulted, is not that
easy to categorize. In part due to his service as surgeon to the
gladiators, he was thoroughly aware of the practical applications
of anatomical and localized thinking. To Galen it was unthink-
able that a surgeon should attack a war wound or remove a bone
without knowing the positions of the nerves, muscles, and blood
vessels involved.

We see, then, that anatomical thinking and its practical arms,
localization of disease and localized treatment, existed throughout the ancient period. Such thinking never was very important,
however. The Greek medical thought that dominated the Middle
Ages in the Latin West would be Galen's humoralism. The conception of disease as localized would not begin to erode the foundation of the doctrine of the four humors until a science of
pathology based on autopsy experience began accumulating. For

our purposes this period can be said to begin with the *anatomia privata* of medieval origin, the private dissections performed to discover the cause of death, particularly where homicide was suspected.

The Beginnings of Pathology

As suggested earlier, the dissection of the human body yields information that is determined in large measure by the questions being asked. In part to prove Vesalius wrong and in part due to the spirit of the time, anatomical dissection increased greatly during and after the sixteenth century. In the first post-Vesalian decades, most of this effort was devoted to understanding normal structure. But the abnormal could not be ignored; anomalies had to be noted if one was to grasp the full range of normality. Diseased organs were encountered as well, and from the fifteenth century on a growing number of men involved themselves in what can be termed pathological investigation. In the fifteenth century the Florentine physician Antonio Benivieni (1443–1502) indicated that it was already common practice for physicians to seek permission to perform autopsies on cases of obscure disease. Benivieni recorded a dozen autopsy reports in which, at times confusedly, he described gallstone, abdominal abscess, and other less certain findings. In 1679 a book appeared bearing the abbreviated title of *Sepulchretum*. The author was the Genevese physician Théophile Bonet (1620–1689), and the book was a massive collection of some three thousand autopsy cases culled from the medical literature of the previous two centuries. Bonet was handicapped by the fact that he was a collector, not an anatomist. Very little of the *Sepulchretum* was tested against his own experience. The book is significant nonetheless, because it demonstrates a dawning realization that autopsy findings can facilitate the understanding of disease.

Even those individuals who were dissecting primarily as anatomists inevitably made contributions to the notion of localized pathology. A prime example here is the Dutch physician Frederik Ruysch (1638–1731), who provides an early glimpse of a process that proved to be amazingly fecund in the later understanding of disease, the exercise now termed clinical-pathological correlation. The correlation involves an attempt to understand the signs and symptoms in living patients by the findings of the post-mortem examination, and Ruysch provides several fine examples of the art. The same technique was exploited by Giovanni Maria Lancisi (1654–1720) and Raymond Vieussens (1635 or 1641 to 1715), when they arrived at a correct understanding, at least in its main features, of the complicated syndrome known as congestive heart failure. Vieussens contributed, as well, what for his time were extraordinarily accurate depictions of hydrothorax (fluid in the chest), hydropericardium (fluid in the heart's sac), and mitral stenosis (a valvular disease of the heart).

It is clear from the writings just described that physicians after 1500 or so were seeing localized manifestations of disease on a regular basis. They were examining brains with localized areas of hemorrhage and arteries that had ballooned out before rupturing. Still, they could not translate the obvious localized alterations in structure to a generalization that the cause of disease itself operated locally. Humoralism remained ascendant. For instruction on this point we can turn to the 1694 report of the autopsy made on the Italian scientist Marcello Malpighi (1628–1694), who had first demonstrated the existence of capillaries, the microscopic connections between arteries and veins. The post-mortem revealed hemorrhage into the right ventricle of the brain, clearly a localized finding. But the *cause* of the hemorrhage was another matter. The dissector, Malpighi's student Giorgio Baglivi (1668–1707), concluded that the necropsy proved that glands in the body had poured into the blood two humors, which when they reached the brain corroded the artery and caused the bleeding. Death was indeed due to hemorrhage, but the hemorrhage came from the corrosive effect of two malign humors, not from disease originating in the artery itself.

Morgagni and Modern Pathology

In the eighteenth century there appeared a man who differed from previous pathologists in much the same way as Vesalius had differed from his predecessors in anatomy. Giovanni Battista Morgagni (1682–1771) was practicing medicine in Forli when, in 1711, he was called to Padua to become assistant professor of theoretical medicine. He labored some fifty years before bringing out his most important book, a studied caution that would not have carried him very far up today's academic ladder. The book describes some seven hundred autopsies, many by his mentor, Valsalva, but the majority executed by himself. The wealth of autopsy material available to Morgagni in eighteenth-century Padua is evidenced not only by the large number of dissections he performed, but by the occupations he gives for his subjects. The usual assortment of strumpets, prostitutes, and mendicants people his pages, but we find also noblemen, nuns, priests, and even a cardinal.

The cases were arranged traditionally, *a capite ad calcem* (head to foot), but they were more than simple autopsy reports. Morgagni demonstrated the immense potential of the process of clinical-pathological correlation. This logical wedding of the signs and symptoms of disease to autopsy findings gradually dispelled all manner of confusion in the classification of disease. It was the basis of the clinical school which would make Paris the medical mecca of the Western world during the first half of the nineteenth century. Two of Morgagni's examples can give the flavor of the whole. A man suffered an aneurysm (ballooning) of the main blood vessel leaving the heart, which finally ruptured, leading to death by exsanguination. After tracing the signs and symptoms that characterized the aneurysm before its fatal outcome, Morgagni described the autopsy findings of a greatly thinned aorta, so enlarged that it had eroded the bones of the anterior chest before it burst.

The second example was a Paduan nun who was suddenly seized by chills and fever. Twenty-four hours later she developed chest pain and a cough. To Morgagni the clinical picture described lobar pneumonia, and he predicted that at the autopsy the affected lung would have the consistency of liver, by which he meant that the normally light, spongy tissue would be solidified and rendered heavy by the localized infection.

This correlating process, repeated hundreds of times, gave Morgagni an unprecedented ability to recognize disease during life and to predict its outcome. He published his life's work in 1761 as *De sedibus et causis morborum* (On the Seats and Causes of Disease), a title which has great significance for our conceptual thread. The book did more than merely demonstrate to physicians the teaching powers of clinical-pathological correlations; it also demonstrated that disease arose from localized changes within the body's organs. The *sedibus* of diseases lay not in the humors that made up the fluid portion of the body but in the solid structure of the organs. Galenic pathology was not to end with Morgagni, but the path of its demise was now laid.

It has been said that Morgagni's seed fell "upon hard and sterile ground," and it is true that no revolution in medical practice ensued immediately after the book was published. But *De sedibus* was reprinted several times in Morgagni's lifetime and was translated into English in 1769, only eight years after its appearance. Clearly the work was being read.

Despite the importance we attach to his efforts, it is apparent that the concept of localized disease was not translated into important changes in the practices of most medical men during Morgagni's lifetime. This is understandable, because, for the bedside physician, localizing the origin of disease offered little significant practical advantage over humoral pathology. What difference did it make if disease originated in the organs? The most important organs in terms of mortality and morbidity—the tripod of life as they have been called—are the brain, heart, and lungs, and these are largely inaccessible to the senses. Other important organs, such as the kidneys, pancreas, and liver, even though not completely hidden behind bony structures, can be seen or felt only when disease is far advanced. What was lacking was a way to extend the senses, improvements in the artful science of physical diagnosis. These innovations were not long arriving, and in retrospect we can see that Morgagni indeed introduced the anatomical idea into the ordinary practice of medicine, that however sterile the ground may have been, his seed survived.

The Rise of Physical Diagnosis

In the eighteenth century the center of bedside teaching was the Dutch city of Leyden. There, under the direction of Herman Boerhaave (1668-1738), an entire generation of students perfected their clinical skills around a mere twelve hospital beds, six devoted to men and six to women. Boerhaave's favorite student, Gerhard van Swieten (1700-1772), was summoned to Vienna in the summer of 1745 by the Empress Maria Theresa, who had not been on the throne long before she realized that the university in Vienna needed a thoroughgoing reform. Through the efforts of van Swieten and his director of the clinic, Anton de Haen (1704–1776), the old Vienna School, as it would later be called, became the model for emulation by many European schools as clinical medicine developed during the eighteenth century.

It was in Vienna, in this atmosphere of clinical excellence, that Leopold Auenbrugger (1722–1809) devised the first of the two important extenders of the physician's senses with which we will be concerned. This was the technique termed percussion, which depends on the fact that tapping the human body over airfilled spaces such as the lungs or an empty stomach results in a resonant note, whereas the same operation over fleshy parts produces a dull sound. The fact is important in disease because the normal lung, for instance, with its myriads of tiny airfilled sacs, renders a resonant note to percussion, but if the sacs are filled with pus, as in pneumonia, the note becomes dull. Awkward and unrefined though the procedure appears to those first learning it, percussion in the hands of an expert can reveal a generous amount of information about the lungs and, to a lesser degree, the heart. Percussion had been practiced on a few occasions before Auenbrugger, but it appears that he was unaware of these earlier halting attempts. A significant aspect of his talent lay in his musical ability. Interpreting the percussion note obviously is enhanced by a good ear. Auenbrugger's musical accomplishments were such that they removed him from the ranks of the strictly amateur; he wrote the libretto for Antonio Salieri's comic opera "The Chimney Sweep." Also important in the story of percussion is that in his childhood he almost certainly observed persons in his father's inn tapping wine casks to determine the level of the liquid therein. He suggests as much in his book, where he makes a direct analogy between tapping a fluid-filled chest and striking a cask containing a fluid.

Auenbrugger labored for seven years perfecting percussion, at times testing his findings by injecting water into the thorax of a dead body. In 1761 he published his small volume, *Inventum novum.* He introduced his "new invention" with seemly modesty, but he had no doubts about the accuracy of his method nor of its value to medicine. From long experience he concluded that many diseases of the chest could be discovered by percussion alone.

Auenbrugger's fate was that of Morgagni, a brief surge of recognition, then eclipse to be followed by rediscovery. We may assume that *Inventum novum* was read by some, as a new edition was issued within two years. But percussion did not spread widely or rapidly among medical practitioners. To Auenbrugger's great distress, the technique was ignored even by the principal clinic in his own Vienna. With few exceptions his contribution languished in obscurity for almost half a century. It was revived in 1808, the year before Auenbrugger died, and eventually became part of a routine physical examination. The importance of the book in the conceptual history of disease is found in Sigerist's words, "It was this same year 1761 that Morgagni's great work was published. The two books were expressions of an identical movement, expressions of the advancing anatomical idea. Morgagni laid the foundations of pathological anatomy, and Auenbrugger laid the foundations of anatomical diagnosis."[1]

Corvisart

To Vienna in the late eighteenth century came a young physician in search of the clinical experience he could not obtain in his home city of Paris. Jean Nicolas Corvisart (1755-1821) qualified as a physician in 1785. His refusal to be shackled by tradition surfaced soon thereafter when he was offered a position in the hospital founded by Mme. Necker but refused when he learned he would have to wear a powdered wig. It was in Vienna that Corvisart learned of the neglected percussion, and for some twenty years he strove to improve on Auenbrugger's method. In 1806 he demonstrated the potential of the technique as applied to the heart in his *Essay on the Diseases and Organic Lesions of the Heart and Great Vessels*. Two years later he recalled Auenbrugger from eclipse, not only translating *Inventum novum*, but enlarging it from 95 to 440 pages through addition from his own rich experience. In an exemplary display of intellectual honesty, Corvisart gave credit where it was due, naming Auenbrugger as the sole originator of percussion.

In Corvisart's hands the combination of precise physical examination, correlated with autopsy findings, was raised to a level of such excellence that it formed the basis of what came to be called the Paris Clinical School. As a means of deriving new medical information, the careful history and physical examination, correlated with autopsy findings, dominated Western medicine for the first half of the nineteenth century. As extended by one of Corvisart's students, Laennec, it came to be known simply as *la méthode,* a distinction it would carry for some one hundred years.

Laennec and the Stethoscope

Percussion has distinct limitations even in the best of hands. The dull note produced by an uncomplicated lobar pneumonia may not be distinguishable from that of fluid between the lung and chest wall due to heart failure or from the consolidation associated with cancer of the bronchus. In part its importance derives from the fact that it came along when physicians had no other available tools but looking, smelling, and feeling. Percussion depended on artificial sounds created by the physician and gave little information about the sounds produced naturally by the heart and lungs in health and disease. An instrument for listening to otherwise inaccessible organs, the stethoscope as it would be called, was contributed by another member of the Paris Clinical School, René Théophile Hyacinthe Laennec (1781–1826).

As a part of the physical examination, Laennec regularly employed a method of listening to the chest known as immediate auscultation, meaning his ear was placed *immediately* over the heart or lungs. This procedure, as Laennec knew, dated back to the Hippocratic physicians, who had described pathological sounds in such phrases as, "It bubbles like boiling vinegar," to describe the fluid in the alveoli, and "It creaks like a new leather strap," for what is now termed a friction rub, the noise resulting when an inflamed lung rubs against the chest wall during respiratory motion. The Greek legacy also included Hippocratic succussion, a sloshing sound heard when a patient with a partially collapsed lung and fluid in the chest cavity is literally shaken to and fro.

Immediate auscultation had serious drawbacks, and these were well known to Laennec. It was inconvenient; it was indelicate in the case of females; and even the hardened physician could have his sensitivity bruised by touching a charity patient, who in those days may well have had his last bath four years earlier when he stumbled out of the *Coq d'Or* and fell into the Seine. Above all, the sounds heard by immediate auscultation were weak and diffuse, and in the case of obese patients, all but inaudible.

The origin of the idea for the stethoscope was recounted in a letter by one of Laennec's friends, who wrote that Laennec had happened to observe children transmitting messages through a long piece of wood by tapping one end with a pin. From this stimulus he rolled up a quire of paper and applied it to a patient's chest, and was surprised that he could hear the heart sounds much more clearly than with his ear directly on the thorax.

Laennec christened his new instrument "stethoscope," from the Greek breast or chest, plus to look or explore. For three years he engaged in *la méthode* – taking a detailed history, performing a thorough physical examination, including auscultation with the new stethoscope, and when death ensued, following the patient to the autopsy table, there to correlate all the findings. In 1819 he published *A Treatise on Mediate Auscultation and on Diseases of the Lungs and Heart.* The title is significant for at least two reasons. The first is the word *mediate,* meaning something interposed between ear and chest. The second relates to his study of diseases of the heart. Auenbrugger's percussion could reveal little about the heart beyond its size. Laennec's stethoscope in effect put the physician inside the heart, where he could hear aberrations in rhythm and the murmurs caused by leaking valves. As one historian put it, "Laennec thereby did more than provide the medical profession with a somewhat more dignified symbol than the medieval urinal; he opened a whole new world for medicine."[2]

That whole new world can perhaps best be illustrated by Laennec's illumination of tuberculosis. For years physicians had been burdened with a murky condition termed phthisis, which at times included tuberculosis but which also embraced any generalized wasting of the body associated with chest symptoms such as cough. Utilizing his new tool, Laennec was able to sort out this welter of lung conditions and for the first time identify phthisis with pulmonary tuberculosis only.

Laennec's book was not doomed to the period of interment that shrouded Auenbrugger's. True, the stethoscope was met with skepticism and ridicule in certain quarters. A segment of the profession simply failed to find any value in the technique, and others feared the dehumanization that such mechanization would bring to the art of medicine. Laennec himself urged his colleagues not to let localized thinking cloud the fact that illness remained at bottom an individual phenomenon.

Scarcely veiled national chauvinism was evident in the assessment of the stethoscope by the man who translated Laennec's book into English.

That it will ever come into general use, notwithstanding its value . . . [is] extremely doubtful; because its beneficial application requires much time and gives a good bit of trouble both to the patient and the practitioner; and because its whole hue and character is foreign, and opposed to all our habits and associations. . . . There is something even ludicrous in the picture of a grave physician formally listening through a long tube applied to the patient's thorax.[3]

This despite the fact that the first English translation was made in 1821, only two years after the original. It is a measure of the slow acceptance of change at the time to recall that when Laennec offered mediate auscultation to the medical world, percussion itself was still almost unknown in England. As it turned out, the doubters were too pessimistic. The stethoscope was accepted widely and relatively rapidly, and before long students were flocking to Paris from as far away as the United States. Because of percussion and the stethoscope, anatomical thinking and its conceptual descendant, disease as localized, had been rendered useful to the average physician in the diagnosis of disease.

Bichat and Tissue Pathology

Morgagni's organ pathology was a fruitful first step in the localization of disease, but clinical experience soon revealed certain deficiencies in the concept. For example, Morgagni's scheme worked well enough in that form of arthritis called gout, in which only one member, such as the big toe, may be afflicted. But what of rheumatoid arthritis, which characteristically involves many joints simultaneously? By this time it was well known to physicians that disease in widely separated organs could at times present the same symptoms. The question now became, how could these findings be squared with the notion that disease originated in the organs?

Medical men also knew by this time that organs were not homogeneous, but rather were composed of different tissues. No microscope was needed to demonstrate this; one has only to cut an organ such as the kidney and discover an outer cortex and inner medulla, or cut the brain, with its distinct layers of gray and white. Some of these tissues are exceedingly widely distributed, fibrous tissue for example, which is present in the coverings of many structures, ranging from the brain to the joints of the foot. Was it possible that disease originated in those tissues rather than in the entire organ? If so, the problem of gout and rheumatoid arthritis would be less perplexing. This was the thesis that would be tested and adopted by another French physician, Marie-François-Xavier Bichat (1771–1802).

Born the son of a country physician, Bichat shared at least two characteristics with Laennec: industriousness and tuberculosis that was finally fatal. By the age of twenty-eight he was chief physician at the famous hospital, *Hôtel Dieu*. His dissecting experience soon led him to conclude that several post-mortems could yield more information than twenty years at the bedside. There is no reason to doubt the depths of his conviction on this score. He reportedly executed some six hundred autopsies in one winter, at times even sleeping in the morgue.

To link disease to certain tissues, Bichat first had to know the tissues of which the organs were composed. This he set out to investigate by gross dissection and by submitting tissues to chemical and physical treatments such as heat, air, water, acids, alkalies, salts, dessication, maceration, putrefaction, and boiling. By these means Bichat arrived at a classification of twenty-one tissues. Combining his system of tissues with many clinical-pathological correlations, Bichat derived a new pathology. His experience drove him to conclude that disease arose not from the compound organs, but from one or more of the organs' tissues which the disease attacked separately. In 1800, two years before his death, Bichat published his evidence and conclusions in a book called *Treatise on Membranes*.

Despite the imperfections of his system of tissues, Bichat's contribution provided a necessary connection to what was coming. He effectively introduced tissues into the science of pathology and, in the process, removed the seat of disease from the organ to the tissue. It was a logical link in the chain of localization, the next being the further refinement that came to be known as cellular pathology.

Virchow and the Cellular Seat of Disease

The same year, 1839, that Theodor Schwann (1810–1882) identified the cell as the basic biological unit of plants and animals, witnessed the arrival in Berlin of the man who would be credited with removing the seat of disease from Bichat's tissue to Schwann's cell. Rudolf Ludwig Carl Virchow (1821–1902) was born in Schivelbein, a small city in Pomerania. In 1843 he took his medical degree under Johannes Mueller (1801–1858), whose gifted students read like a *Who's Who* of nineteenth-century German biological science. As early as 1845 Virchow agreed with Schwann that the cell was the fundamental unit of the body. At that point he also shared Schwann's belief that cells arose from a formless substance called the blastema, an encumberment Virchow had to escape before he could develop fully his thesis that the cell is the basic unit of disease.

The question of inflammation and pus formation can illustrate the major differences between the blastema theory and that of cellular pathology. As Virchow arrived on the scene, the traditional wisdom explained pus formation along the following lines. The smallest blood vessels gradually narrow down to the point that the blood is finally greatly slowed. There follows a process called exudation, in which the blastema oozes through the intact wall of the tiny blood vessels. From this blastema, cells form along the lines described by Schwann, and these are the pus cells or fibrous cells of the scar, which are then observable by the microscope. Our present conception of pus formation is altogether different, holding that the pre-existing white blood cells migrate to the site of inflammation and extrude themselves actively through the blood vessel wall in a process known as diapedesis.

It was Virchow's contribution to destroy the whole notion of the blastema. In its stead he established the concept of *omnis cellula a cellula,* that all cells come from pre-existing cells. The ramifications of this proved far reaching indeed. Scientists and physicians would now look at disease from a completely new point of view. Diseased cells would be thought of not as new, but as modifications of previously normal cells. The importance of the difference is easily perceived when looked at in the instance of cancer. If cancer cells arose *de novo,* it would be impossible to assign a given malignant tissue to an organ, that is, to distinguish between cancer of the breast and that of the lung by similarities between normal and cancerous cells. But if all cells came from pre-existing cells, it would be possible to trace cancer cells back to their normal precursors and then search for the influences that had converted them from benign to malignant. For Virchow, then, all cells had to come from existing cells, and the cell became the locus of disease as well.

In assessing Virchow's contributions, we can begin by saying what has been said before, but what cannot be emphasized too often in a survey of the present sort. He had forerunners in all of his major contributions to medicine. He was not even the first to maintain the continuity of cellular life. It has been concluded that the principle of *omnis cellula a cellula* was actually "developed" by Robert Remak (1815–1865) and only further "formulated" by Virchow. August Foerster (1822–1865) must be mentioned as well, because in 1855 he reached essentially identical conclusions to those Virchow would enunciate in definitive form a few years later.

Nor did Virchow alone originate cellular pathology. He put forth his ideas on the subject in a paper in 1855 and his more famous elaboration in a book three years later. But in 1852 Remak had already concluded that pathological tissues did not originate in the blastema, but came from normal forerunners instead. Virchow is honored as the founder of cellular pathology, then, not because he alone conceived it, but rather because of the evidence he garnered in its support and the system he devised and perfected for its use in diagnosing and understanding disease. Our purpose does not demand a complete analysis of his accomplishments and errors. The seat of the disease had moved once again, this time to the cellular level, and the major credit for this achievement belongs to Rudolf Virchow.

Localized Disease and Surgery

Our story began on the river of the anatomical idea, branched into the concept of localized disease, and then took another tributary to discover how anatomical thinking came to be useful to practicing physicians through advances in physical diagnosis. In concluding this segment of the story, it remains to look in passing at localized thinking and the practices of surgery.

For most of history surgeons knew the hazards of operating within the body's cavities. It was only after generalized anesthesia and antisepsis became available in the nineteenth century that surgeons began invading the abdomen, thorax, and skull with relative impunity. For centuries, then, with rare exceptions, surgical practice was limited to such procedures as amputations, cataract removal, repair of hernias, dental extractions, removal of bladder stones from below, and excision of tumors of skin, muscles, and bone. A moment's reflection makes it apparent that the operations just listed involve a localized approach to diagnosis and treatment. An aching tooth, a boil, a gangrenous foot, a spurting artery, all are overwhelmingly localized by their very nature and naturally suggest extraction, lancing, amputation, and ligature. The urgency of such conditions, plus the obviousness of their treatment, have led historians to discover the origins of surgery in the human instinct and to postulate the beginnings of Greek medicine as deriving from surgery. This is also why it does not surprise us to discover that, long before Morgagni, surgeons were perforce thinking and operating at the localized level.

If we agree that the conditions amenable to the knife demanded a localized approach to diagnosis and cure, the question arises, what kept the localized thinking of surgeons from spilling over into and influencing medicine at large? The assumed answer has been that the split that existed for much of Western history between the low-caste barber-surgeon and the academic surgeon who did not operate, and the further overall split between surgeons and physicians, did not permit much in the way of intellectual cross-fertilization. As it turns out, the answer is not so simple.

Soon after the medieval universities began developing in the thirteenth century, medicine came to be classified as a science, while surgery was designated as a technical discipline. Under this arrangement physicians assumed the role of directing surgeons, and since this demanded a certain amount of theorization, surgeons were gradually subdivided into academic surgeons and a lower, uneducated group characterized as barber-surgeons. This split was to persist into the modern period, the educational system underpinning the schism, in some places surviving well into the seventeenth century. Although social and legal barriers were guaranteed to perpetuate the cleavage between physicians and surgeons, and among the surgeons themselves, it is known now that the two groups were not as thoroughly separated in practice as might be supposed.

The evolution of surgery in France illustrates the difficulties surgeons had in liberating their specialty from its medieval heritage. For centuries the three contending parties were the physicians of the *École de Médicine,* the academic surgeons or surgeons of the long robe, and the barbers (surgeons of the short robe). Between 1655 and 1660 the surgeons and barbers were effectively merged. From this lowly assignation the surgeons slowly struggled to regain a professional respect, aided along the way by Louis XIV and Louis XV. Largely through the influence of Georges Mareschal (1658-1736), who went from an uneducated and penniless apprentice-surgeon to become *premier chirurgien du Roi,* surgery was removed from the domination of the Faculty of Medicine by an act of *Parlement* in 1724. In 1731 the Royal Academy of Surgery was created, and in 1743 the surgeons were separated from the barbers and their practice regulated. The King was persuaded in this latter by François de la Peyronie (1678-1747), a prominent Montpellier surgeon who had joined Mareschal in founding the Academy of Surgery. Thus it was that Paris became a surgical center in the eighteenth century. Into this now generally benign environment came Pierre-Joseph Desault (1738-1795), whose inspirational leadership would set the stage for the final elevation of surgery to parity with medicine.

Desault's contribution was his perfection of what was called the surgical lesson, a close variant of the clinical-pathological correlation just discussed. In addition to a detailed account of the patient's history, physical examination, and clinical course, the report included an autopsy, wherein the surgeons attempted to localize the disease as well as discover its nature. The connection to what has gone before in this discussion relates to the fact that both Corvisart and Bichat were students of Desault. Also now rendered comprehensible is the comment by Laennec, in the preface to the 1826 second edition of his famous book, to the effect that his principal goal was to place medical diagnosis on the same level as that of surgical diagnosis. At a time when European physicians generally considered themselves vastly superior to surgeons, Laennec here informs us that in the arena of diagnosis, at least, the surgical method deserved emulation. It is now evident that a number of accepted notions concerning the historical split between medicine and surgery have been consistently exaggerated or misconstrued. More recent investigations provide documentation for what common sense might have led us to believe, that the nature of surgical lesions has always predisposed to localized thinking and that such thinking, at various times and places, although most demonstrably in the Paris Clinical School and thereafter, influenced ideas of medical thought generally.

Epilogue

The cell, of course, was not the end. The ascendancy of the cell theory and cellular pathology, as is often true of major developments in the history of disease, raised as many questions as they answered. Here we need make only the single point that the process of reseating the origin of disease in ever finer structures continues in our time. The term molecular pathology was coined sometime before 1945, and its science can be said to date back at least to 1948, when an abnormal hemoglobin was determined as the cause of sickle cell anemia. Despite Virchow's lamentation that molecular properties, while necessary, would remain an insufficient explanation of the life processes of the cell, the mechanistic approach continued to attract most biologists.

The trend seems destined to continue. Atomic diseases are now recognized, and there is a specialty known as nuclear medicine. All of this brings the historian perilously close to the pitfalls of contemporary history, but the phenomenon must be mentioned at least to avoid the notion that the work of one man, regardless of its excellence, ends a given concept of disease by exploiting it fully. Virchow established to everyone's satisfaction that all cells come from pre-existing cells. A century later there is evidence that certain pathogens, mycoplasms and viruses, may actually originate *de novo*. On more than one occasion, the conceptual history of disease has developed more in the nature of a circle than of a series of blocks aligned unidirectionally in time.

Notes

1. Sigerist, H. E. *The Great Doctors.* New York: Dover Publications, 1971, p. 241.
2. Ackerknecht, E. H. *A Short History of Medicine.* New York: Ronald Press Company, 1968, p. 151.
3. Laennec, R.T.H. *A Treatise on the Disease of the Chest,* John Forbes, tr. New York: Hafner Publishing Company, 1962, p. xix.

Bibliographic Commentary

Our understanding of localized thinking about disease in antiquity has been enhanced by the exchange between W. D. Smith, "Galen on Coans versus Cnidians," *Bull. Hist. Med.* 47:569-585, 1973, and I. M. Lonie, "Cos versus Cnidus and the Historians," parts 1 and 2, *Hist. Sci.* 16:42-75, 77-92, 1978. My description of Cnidian pathology follows Lonie, "The Cnidian Treatises of the *Corpvs Hippocraticvm,"* *Classical Quarterly,* n.s. 15:1-3, 1965. Evidence of Galen's localism is derived from G.E.R. Lloyd, *Greek Science After Aristotle,* London: Chatto & Windus, 1973.

Renaissance developments in pathology are covered by E. R. Long, *A History of Pathology,* New York: Dover Publications, 1965, and *Selected Readings in Pathology,* Springfield, Ill.: Charles C. Thomas, 1961.

The evolution of our understanding of congestive heart failure is told in a model of research in the history of clinical medicine by S. Jarcho, *The Concept of Heart Failure: From Avicenna to Albertini,* Cambridge: Harvard University Press, 1980. Morgagni's case studies are from *The Seats and Causes of Diseases,* translated by W. Cooke, Boston: Wells and Lilly and H. C. Carey and I. Lea, 1824. Although more detailed studies exist, a beginner's interest in the Old Vienna School will be satisfied by E. Lesky, "The Development of Bedside Teaching at the Vienna Medical School from Scholastic Times to Special Clinics," in C. D. O'Malley, ed., *The History of Medical Education,* Berkeley: University of California Press, 1970. Lesky treats the later years in *The Vienna Medical School of the Nineteenth Century,* Baltimore: Johns Hopkins University Press, 1976.

The most useful English translation of Auenbrugger is by J. Forbes, in *Inventum Novum,* London: Dawsons of Pall Mall, 1966. This edition also contains a facsimile of the first edition, the French and German translations by J. N. Corvisart and S. Ungar respectively, and a short biographical sketch in German by M. Neuburger. Also valuable is H. Sigerist's introduction to Forbes's translation in *Bull.*

Institute Hist. Med. 4:373–377, 1936. There is an English translation by J. Gates of
J. N. Corvisart's *An Essay on the Organic Diseases and Lesions of the Heart and
Great Vessels,* New York: Hafner, 1962.

A partial translation by J. Forbes of Laennec's *magnum opus* is reprinted in
C.N.B. Camac, *Classics of Medicine and Surgery,* New York: Dover Publications,
1959. A more complete version by the same translator appears as *A Treatise on
the Diseases of the Chest,* New York: Hafner Publishing Company, 1962.

The definitive treatment of the Paris Clinical School is that by E. H. Ackerknecht, *Medicine at the Paris Hospital, 1794–1848,* Baltimore: Johns Hopkins University Press, 1967.

Two of Bichat's three most important books have English translations, but
unfortunately not the *Traité des membranes.*

Virchow's medical thought is explored by L. J. Rather in his fine introduction to
R. Virchow, *Cellular Pathology,* translated by F. Chance, New York: Dover Publi-
cations, 1971. Also valuable in this regard, but particularly in its objective assess-
ment of Virchow's contributions, is E. H. Ackerknecht, *Rudolf Virchow: Doctor,
Statesman, Anthropologist,* Madison: University of Wisconsin Press, 1953. The
importance of distinguishing normal cells from abnormal is nicely elucidated by
L. J. Rather, *The Genesis of Cancer: A Study in the History of Ideas,* Baltimore:
Johns Hopkins University Press, 1978.

My account of the evolution of French surgery follows T. Gelfand, *Professionalizing Modern Medicine: Paris Surgeons and Medical Science and Institutions in the
Eighteenth Century,* Westport, Conn.: Greenwood Press, 1980, and the analysis of
the importance of surgery in localized thinking derives from the seminal paper
by O. Temkin, "The Role of Surgery in the Rise of Modern Medical Thought," *The
Double Face of Janus,* Baltimore: Johns Hopkins University Press, 1977.

The extrapolation of localized pathology beyond the cell is pursued by E. L.
Hess, "Origins of Molecular Biology," *Science* 168:664–669, 1970.

7
THE CONCEPT OF EXPERIMENTAL MEDICINE

Strictly speaking, the conceptual history of disease could be written without a chapter on experimental medicine. Such a product, however, would leave a large and possibly confusing hiatus. In 1870 physicians could do little to cure or prevent disease. A hundred years later they could intervene tellingly in many of mankind's more important diseases. In a single century the understanding of disease increased more than in the previous forty centuries combined. The two crucial developments in this regard were the rise of technology and the application of the basic biological sciences to medicine, using new rules of experimentation and new criteria of proof. Without some understanding of the rapid development of these instruments in the last half of the nineteenth and first half of the twentieth centuries, the student of medical history would have difficulty comprehending the remarkable advances in the understanding of disease and the ability to control it which have taken place during the last century.

With Virchow the anatomical idea was extended to the study of disease as it produced structural changes within the cell. Virchow and his critics hoped that his "pathology of the future" would embrace not merely changes in *structure* but also pathological physiology, that is, changes in the *function* of cells as a result of disease. As it turned out, cellular pathology developed narrowly along anatomical lines, as Virchow himself finally admitted in 1898. And just as cellular pathology had to be built on a knowledge of normal cells (histology), pathological physiology would await a greater understanding of normal function. This is the body of knowledge that accrued to investigators plying the artistic science of experimental medicine.

An experiment consists of putting a question to nature and interpreting the response. Properly done it is a far more rigorous exercise than many imagine. The current medical literature abounds in examples of experiments which, because of faulty design, could never answer the question being asked. For years physicians treated victims of heart attack (myocardial infarction) with drugs that decreased the blood's ability to clot. Periodically they reported their experiences in medical journals, the number of cases finally exceeding 10,000. Despite this mountain of clinical experience, doubts persisted about whether anticoagulant therapy prevented future heart attacks. When two scientists finally analyzed the thirty-two papers containing the 10,000 patient reports, not one experiment met all the standards necessary to yield the greatest possible useful information.

The nonscientist might be inclined to criticize the example just cited, but practicing scientists would be more understanding. The pitfalls in medical experimentation are numerous and at times difficult to anticipate. Several years ago it was discovered that cancer of the cervix was rare in Jewish women. Some resourceful investigator concluded that circumcision in their husbands somehow protected women against this form of cancer. To verify his hypothesis he questioned a group of women who had cervical cancer and found that indeed a high proportion of their husbands were uncircumcised. A second investigator doubted if women always knew whether their husbands were circumcised and so asked the husbands instead. He found a somewhat higher incidence of circumcised men than that reported in the first study. A third scientist doubted whether husbands *or* wives would always have accurate information on the question at hand, so had the husbands examined by a physician. This investigator found very little correlation between cervical cancer and circumcision, but did discover frequent disagreement between wives, husbands, and physicians as to whether circumcision had in fact been done. To put the matter to rest, a fourth study had two physicians independently examine the husbands, but this too ended up in defeat; the physicians themselves frequently disagreed over the presence or absence of circumcision. Thus what appeared in theory to be a rather simple question turned out in practice to be insoluble given the method employed. A scientist cannot compare items unless he can delimit them precisely, and in biological systems this first necessary step can be difficult to traverse. A pregnancy is always a pregnancy, but a circumcision is not always a circumcision.

It is beyond the scope of this chapter to recount the full development of the concept of experimental medicine. Rather, three eras will be sampled in an attempt to give some understanding of the growing sophistication of experimental medicine as anatomical knowledge and thinking became more important in medical thought. There will be a look at an experiment by Galen in second-century Rome, then one by William Harvey in seventeenth-century England, and finally a somewhat longer consideration of the work and experimental philosophy of Claude Bernard in nineteenth-century France.

Galen and the Formation of Urine

Although his technology was limited largely to his knife, Galen staged a number of physiological demonstrations that can only be termed elegant. In animals he severed the spinal cord and showed the resultant loss of motion and sensibility. Performing before some of the great names of Rome, he silenced a pig by ligating its laryngeal nerve and returned the animal's squeal by releasing the ligature. One of his more impressive experiments was his proof that urine is formed by the kidneys and transmitted to the bladder by the ureters. Galen began his description of this phase of his work by examining the theory of urine formation espoused by Asclepiades, who had come to Rome in the first century B.C. and who helped raise Greek physicians to the dominance they came to enjoy in the new center of the Western world. In Galen's words, Asclepiades believed that "the fluid which we drink passes into the bladder by being resolved into vapours, and that, when these have been again condensed, it thus regains its previous form, and turns from vapour into liquid." In short, urine formed inside the bladder by a process resembling condensation, and little attention was paid to the anatomical relationship between kidney, ureter, and bladder. To put an end to such "nonsensical talk," Galen proceeded in this way:

Now the method of demonstration is as follows. One has to divide the peritoneum in front of the ureters, then secure these with ligatures, and next, having bandaged up the animal, let him go (for he will not continue to urinate). After this, one loosens the external bandages and shows the bladder empty and the ureters quite full and distended – in fact almost on the point of rupturing; on removing the ligature from them, one then plainly sees the bladder becoming filled with urine.

When this has been made quite clear, then, before the animal urinates, one has to tie a ligature round his penis and then to squeeze the bladder all over; still nothing goes back through the ureters to the kidneys. Here, then, it becomes obvious that not only in a dead animal, but in one which is still living, the ureters are prevented from receiving back the urine from the bladder. These observations having been made, one now loosens the ligature from the animal's penis and allows him to urinate, then again ligatures one of the ureters and leaves the other to discharge into the bladder. Allowing, then, some time to elapse, one now demonstrates that the ureter which was ligatured is obviously full and distended on the side next to the kidneys, while the other one – that from which the ligature had been taken – is itself flaccid, but has filled the bladder with urine. Then, again one must divide the full ureter, and demonstrate how the urine spurts out of it, like blood in the operation of venesection; and after this one cuts through the other also, and both being thus divided, one bandages up the animal externally. Then when enough time seems to have elapsed, one takes off the bandages; the bladder will now be found empty, and the whole region between the intestines and the peritoneum full of urine, as if the animal were suffering from dropsy. Now, if anyone will but test this for himself on an animal, I think he will strongly condemn the rashness of Asclepiades.

In this experiment Galen forcefully demonstrated the importance of anatomical considerations in understanding the function of the body's structures. The transition back and forth between anatomical and physiological thinking was for him entirely natural, and he was at times scornful of those who ignored anatomical relationships, saying on one occasion, "Practically every butcher is aware of this, from the fact that he daily observes both the position of the kidneys and the duct (termed the ureter) which runs from each kidney into the bladder, and from this he infers their characteristic use and faculty."[1]

Galen showed that an excellent and resourceful mind could go a long way toward understanding physiology, at least in a gross sense, without the technology and quantification we associate with physiological experimentation today. But, as noted earlier, Galen's lead in experimental medicine was not pursued by the physicians who followed him. Instead, his humoral pathology and therapeutics were taken as the sum of what practitioners needed to know for the day-to-day practice of medicine. To pick up the story of experimental medicine, we leap some fourteen hundred years ahead to a man whose principal contribution would be the correction of one of Galen's more important mistakes.

William Harvey and the Circulation of the Blood

It has been said that anyone who had studied in Padua, the mecca of anatomical study, likely would think in anatomical terms the rest of his life. So it was with William Harvey (1578–1657) who, after preparation at Cambridge, journeyed to Padua where he was awarded his medical degree in 1602. One of Harvey's Paduan teachers was Girolamo Fabrici d'Acquapendente (1537–1619), whose discovery of the valves of the veins would later play a role in Harvey's thought as he pondered the movement of the blood.

As the seventeenth century began, Galen's conception of the motion of the blood dominated medical thinking. In this system, the blood did not circulate as we now know it does. Indeed, by Harvey's time Galen's influence had effectively removed the blood's motion from any further direct experimental study. This was because of the then generally held conviction that the only methods suitable for studying the motion of the blood, such as ligatures and severing of the vessels, were the cause of whatever movement was subsequently observed. One of the more enduring errors describing Galen's idea of the blood's movement is that the motion was one of ebb and flow. We now understand that for Galen the principal movement of the blood was forward; only a negligible amount of blood could reverse its usual direction of flow. Food became blood in the liver, and from there part of the blood went directly to the body by way of the veins, while the rest traveled to the right side of the heart. Here there was a further division, with a small portion going to the lungs and the rest passing to the left side of the heart through the pores which, it may be remembered, Vesalius was unable to find. From the left side of the heart the blood moved out into the body, including the brain. It should be noted that since Galen did not allow for circulation as such, blood had to be formed as rapidly as it was utilized. It was this aspect of Galen's theory that Harvey would attack quantitatively.

Harvey published his explication of the movement of the heart and blood in 1628 as *Exercitatio anatomica de motu cordis et sanguinis in animalibus,* or as it is usually called, *De motu cordis* (On the Motion of the Heart). Formerly historians believed that by 1616 he was convinced that the blood circulated, but this is now generally discounted, and we are left with a later but uncertain date for his final conclusion. The origin of Harvey's theory is also a matter of differing opinion. The usual story, also generally now discounted, is that he got onto the notion of the circulation of the blood while pondering the fact that the venous valves discovered by Fabrici directed the blood toward the heart, which in itself refuted one aspect of Galen's system. Another suggestion is that the necessity for a circulatory motion occurred to Harvey because he found the same blood in the arteries as the veins, meaning there had to be some communication between the two types of vessels. What does seem certain is that he made up his mind that the blood had to circulate before he set about gathering experimental proof for his belief. In this he was heavily influenced by a fundamental conception of natural philosophy at the time, the perfection of circular movement.

Before turning to Harvey's work and a summary of his influence, the discontinuity suggested by a conceptual approach to history should be ameliorated by at least passing mention of his predecessors. As early as the thirteenth century certain aspects of the pulmonary (lesser) circulation were laid out by the Arabic physician Ibn an-Nafīs (ca. 1210–1280). There is evidence that this work was unknown to the Spanish heretic Michael Servetus (1509/1511–1553), when he described the lesser circulation again some three hundred years later. Servetus buried his conclusion in a religious tract, and since his works were suppressed after he was burned at the stake, it has been suggested that his description also had little impact on later thinking. Realdus Columbus (ca. 1510–1559) in 1559 published the first "effective" account of the lesser circulation. Andreas Cesalpinus (1519?–1603), the other man usually mentioned in this regard, added little to what was already accepted. One of the major obstacles Harvey had to face was the tendency of his Renaissance forebears to attribute their observations on the circulation of the blood to abnormal rather than normal functions. Cesalpinus, for example, was able to convince himself that the same blood that moved outward during waking hours returned by way of invisible connections to the veins during sleep, but still thought the usual movement of venous blood was outward.

The priority fight over the discovery of the circulation of the blood has been long and at times bitter. For our purposes it is enough to agree that it was Harvey who put forth a consolidated theory of the circulation of the blood backed by experimental evidence which few could deny. It has been aptly said that Harvey was great not because he discovered the circulation but because he demonstrated it; his method was his contribution.

The details of Harvey's experiments are too lengthy to be reproduced here, although it is amusing in passing to see how adamantly he disposed of Galen's interventricular pores. "But damme," he said, "there are no pores and it is not possible to show such."[2] Rather than survey all of Harvey's experimental evidence, we will focus on his use of quantitative measures, a major contribution, and one that was employed increasingly in physiological work after he demonstrated its potential. In Chapter 9 Harvey put forth three propositions which for him confirmed the main thesis he had developed to that point.

First, the blood is incessantly transmitted by the action of the heart from the vena cava to the arteries in such quantity that it cannot be supplied from the ingesta, and in such wise that the whole must very quickly pass through the organ; second, blood under the influence of the arterial pulse enters and is impelled in a continuous, equable, and incessant stream through every part and member of the body, in much larger quantity than were sufficient for nutrition, or than the whole mass of fluids could supply; third, the veins in like manner return this blood incessantly to the heart from parts and members of the body.[3]

To convince himself of these essentially quantitative statements, Harvey measured the capacity of the heart's chambers and then calculated how much blood the heart could expel into the arteries in a fixed time. His measurements were far from sophisticated, but for his purposes extreme accuracy was not needed. If 1 oz. of blood was discharged with each heart beat, then 83 lb. 4 oz. would enter the arteries each half hour. The damage this did to common sense, Harvey went on to point out, was well known even to butchers, who knew that when they cut the throat of an ox, all the blood escaped within a quarter of an hour.

Quantification in physiological experimentation was not invented by Harvey. Galen himself at one point observed that the amount of urine formed each day must equal the fluid intake less that passed in feces, sweat, and insensible perspiration. Even though quantitative thinking was unusual in Greek physiology, it is possible that Galen influenced Harvey in this regard. Further, it should be remembered that Harvey probably would not have extended his quantitative ruminations to the idea of circulation if he had not been influenced by a variety of other factors, some theoretical and philosophical, others based on his medical beliefs and experiences.

Confirmation of the circulation of the blood had immediate implications for medical theory and practice. In terms of theory, the spread of poisons and "contagions" became understandable. The offending substances of syphilis and rabies were now understood to spread from the chancre or the dog bite by way of the circulating blood. Harvey himself saw the practical potential of his discovery when he reportedly advocated placing a ligature above a poison dart wound and immediately amputating the limb as a means of saving the victim's life. And of course blood transfusions and intravenous medications now at least made theoretical sense and were soon tried, even though their effective application was almost three hundred years in the future.

One final aspect of Harvey's work should be mentioned. Galen, as we have seen, could save his theory only by resorting to pores in the septum of the heart. For postulating what he could not actually see, he has at times been deprecated. Harvey faced a similar impasse and solved it in much the same way. His scheme required the blood to pass from arteries to veins, but the capillaries that form this connection were not discovered until 1661. Harvey concluded that the passages must exist, even though he could not demonstrate them. For this he has been acclaimed on grounds that he was daring in his use of logic. Harvey's leap is more useful for us insofar as it underscores the insufficiency of evaluating historical figures and achievements purely in terms of the way they agree with our current perception of scientific truth. Galen's pores were no less logical for his system merely because they were later found to be nonexistent. And at the time, Harvey's postulated arteriovenous passages were not more scientifically accurate merely because later they turned out to be there.

Claude Bernard

The name of Claude Bernard (1813-1878) is inseparably linked to the concept of experimental medicine. For some the two are all but synonymous, although Bernard probably would have objected to any such easy association. He, more than most, recognized the timelessness of experimental medicine, that the elements of biological investigation were present in the uncontrolled empiricism that characterized most medical innovation before him. But there are painters and there are artists, carpenters and craftsmen, violinists and virtuosos. Bernard did not originate experimental medicine, but he carried it to unprecedented heights, and after him, few doubted the potential of biological science in ferreting out natural truth in living organisms.

In his medical studies Bernard came under the influence of François Magendie (1783-1855), who had replaced Bichat's vitalistic physiology with a strongly deterministic orientation. In 1841 Magendie selected Bernard as an assistant, and the young man thus permanently switched from the track of medical practice to that of biological investigation. His physiological investigations were not science for its own sake, but from the outset reflected a distinct medical orientation. Beginning with his doctoral thesis (1843), which concerned itself with the role of gastric juice in nutrition, and throughout his later work (for example, his thorough discussion of the glycogenic function of the liver which appeared in his book on diabetes), Bernard's experiments had direct implications for clinical medicine.

Once again it is not necessary to detail all of Bernard's contributions to the field of experimental medicine. Rather the focus will be one discovery – the elucidation of sugar in the animal economy. From this phase of Bernard's work it is possible to illustrate his philosophy of experimentation, his method, which, as with Harvey, was perhaps his greatest legacy.

As Bernard began his work on animal sugar, two relevant influential ideas existed. First, it was held that animals could break down (catabolyze) foodstuffs but could not anabolize or build them up. Second, although Magendie had apparently cast some doubt on the notion, it was also believed that sugar appeared in the blood only in pathological conditions such as diabetes. Equipped now with a more sensitive test, Bernard was able to demonstrate that sugar existed normally in the blood, and at this point he made a surprising discovery. Not only could he detect sugar normally in the blood, he found the substance no matter whether the animal was fed carrots, starch, or meat, or even if it had fasted for two days. Where was the sugar coming from? Bernard set out to solve the mystery and in his words, "after some groping which I believe is useless to report here, I was led to search for the source of the sugar" in the abdominal organs. He encountered a good deal of adversity before he determined that blood entering the liver gave a negative test for sugar while that coming from the liver was positive. Further, an analysis of the abdominal organs revealed that the liver alone contained sugar, so that he was now able to conclude that "it was from the liver that the sugar was issuing."

The larger question remained: How was the blood sugar level maintained during periods of sugar fasting? Bernard solved this by demonstrating that the liver stored sugar as a substance which had properties similar to starch, a substance he named glycogen, which the liver released to the blood as needed. The liver, he could now generalize, is "at the same time both the *source* and the *origin* of the saccharine material in animals."[4]

Bernard extrapolated his investigations into one of the most influential physiologic principles in the history of experimental medicine. The body has, as it were, a fluid internal environment which mediates between the external environment and the cells. This is necessary because the delicate intracellular molecules cannot survive direct exposure to the harsh external environment. Thus oxygen is delivered to the body's cells by way of the blood and extracellular fluid at the same time that waste products such as carbon dioxide move through the same channels in the opposite direction. With this conception Bernard balanced Virchow's emphasis on the anatomical approach to understanding the malfunctions we term disease. The body's fluids and the cells were each important in their own way. The life processes went on within the anatomical unit, the cell. For its part the blood not only nurtured the cell and carried away waste products, but mediated one cell's effects on another. With this and other concepts, there was now a rational basis for understanding the mechanism of, say, the endocrine glands. The thyroid cells secrete thyroxine, which has a regulatory effect on the metabolism of other cells in the body, and the thyroxine reaches these other cells by way of the blood, the entire scheme being directed by the nervous system.

Bernard coined the term *milieu intérieur* to denote his internal environment. The idea was extended in 1928, when Walter Cannon devised the concept of homeostasis to indicate the steady state that characterizes the animal organism. Once again, as always, the idea itself was not new. In the seventeenth century the philosopher Spinoza is quoted as having said, "The fundamental principle is the innate tendency of the body to perpetuate its being." But Bernard had proved it by showing it in operation, and therein lies a very large difference.

In the early 1860s Bernard suffered a siege of illness which caused him to return to the region of his birth. There he brought together what might be called his philosophy of physiological investigation. The work was recognized instantly as a classic and led to Bernard's admission to the Academy of France in 1868. He called his book *An Introduction to the Study of Experimental Medicine,* and the fact that it was still read in 1957 as part of the philosophy program in French schools is testimony to both its intellectual content and its literary excellence. L. J. Henderson has given us a paragraph that captures the essence of Bernard's method and thus deserves quotation at length.

The experiment . . . is always undertaken in view of a preconceived idea, but it matters not whether this idea is vague or clearly defined, for it is but the question, vague or otherwise, which he puts to nature. Now, when nature replies, he holds his peace, takes note of the answer, listens to the end and submits to the decision. In short, the experiment is always devised with the help of a working hypothesis; the resulting observation is always made without preconceived idea. Such habits are not too easily formed, for man is by nature proud and inclined to metaphysics, but the practice of experimentation will cure these faults.[5]

A genuine understanding of Bernard's method demands a reading of *Experimental Medicine* in its entertaining and enlightening entirety. A synoptic appreciation may be attainable from applying an outline of his method to one of his actual experiments, the approach that Bernard himself exploits in Part 3 of his book.

THE EXPERIMENTAL METHOD

A. Begins with one of two forms of observation
   1. Planned
   2. Chance (serendipity), which leads to a
B. Hypothesis
   From there the process proceeds identically to
C. Experiment, which must be
   1. Controlled (all variables accounted for)
   2. Reproducible under the same circumstances, followed by
D. Application of counterproof; then
E. Results may be extended to a general proposition or lead to a new hypothesis followed by new experimentation.

The outline, numbers, and letters are not Bernard's. To assist the reader who is unfamiliar with the experimental process, they have been inserted into Bernard's following account of the way in which a chance observation led him to his work on the role of pancreatic juice in digestion. It is, so to speak, an experiment in applying the theory of experimentation to one of Bernard's idealized experiments.

One day rabbits were brought to my laboratory from the market. These were placed on a table where they urinated, and, by chance, I observed [A-2] that their urine was clear and acid. This fact struck me because rabbits, which are herbivores, ordinarily have turbid and alkaline urine, whereas carnivores, as we know, have clear and acid urine. This observation of acid urine in the rabbits suggested that they must be in a nutritional state of carnivores. I supposed that they had not eaten for some time and had been transformed by fasting into veritable carnivores, in effect living on their own blood [B]. Nothing was easier than to verify this preconceived idea by experiment. I fed the rabbits grass and a few hours later their urine was turbid and alkaline [C]. I then subjected them to fasting and within twenty-four to thirty-six hours, their urine was again clear and strongly acid; then after eating grass their urine became alkaline again, etc. [C-1]. I repeated this experiment many times, always with the same result. Then I repeated the process on a horse, an herbivore which also had turbid and alkaline urine. I found that fasting promptly produced acidity of the urine, just as it had in rabbits. . . . [C-1, C-2]. As a result of my experiments I thus reached the general proposition, which was unknown at the time, that all fasting animals feed on meat, so that herbivores develop urine resembling that of carnivores [E],

We are dealing here with a very simple fact which allows us to follow experimental reasoning. When we see an unaccustomed phenomenon, we must always ask ourselves what led to it, or put another way, what is its immediate cause; the answer that occurs to us [B] must then be tested by experimentation [C]. When I saw acid urine in the rabbits, I asked myself instinctively, what the cause could be. The experimental idea consisted in the connection which my mind made spontaneously between the acidity of the rabbits' urine and the fasting state which I considered the same as a carnivorous diet. The inductive reasoning which I implicitly undertook produced the following syllogism: the urine of carnivores is acid; my rabbits have acid urine; therefore they are carnivores, which is to say, fasting [B]. This remained to be verified by experimentation.[C].

But to prove that my rabbits truly were carnivores, a counter-proof was needed. I had to produce a carnivorous rabbit by feeding it meat to see if its urine would become clear and acid as it does during fasting. So I fed the rabbits cold boiled beef (which they eat quite readily if they have nothing else). My expectation was verified again; as long as the meat diet was continued, the rabbits exhibited clear acid urine [D].[6]

Serendipity

Chance, or the refined version of it known as serendipity, played such a recurring role in Bernard's experimentation that it deserves a passing glance. The word serendipity is credited to Horace Walpole, who picked it up after reading "a silly fairy tale, called the Three Princes of Serendip: as their Highnesses travelled, they were always making discoveries, by accidents and sagacity, of things which they were not in quest of."[7]

Without reviewing all of Bernard's work from the standpoint of chance, it is clear that serendipity played a prominent part in many of his experiments, a fact which Bernard freely admitted. "Experimental ideas," he wrote, "are often born by chance; with the help of some casual observation. Nothing is more common; and this is really the simplest way of beginning a piece of scientific work."[8]

He did indeed demonstrate that nothing is more common. Upon opening the abdomen of a rabbit which had been fed fatty food, he noticed that only a portion of the vessels draining the small intestine contained the whitish chyle that represents saponified fats. By observing that the pancreatic duct entered the intestine lower in rabbits than in the dogs he was accustomed to, he was led to his conclusion that pancreatic juice was instrumental in the digestion of fats. There was a further element of chance impinging on the same observation; German physiologists who attempted to duplicate Bernard's findings determined that the unusual distribution of chyle which had caught Bernard's attention was only present if the rabbit was opened at the proper time after the test meal was given.

His chance observation that blood in a renal vein was bright red when the organ was actively secreting, and dark red when the organ was more or less at rest, led him to conclude that the secretory function of certain glands is under nervous control. His determination that diabetes (increased blood sugar) could be produced by obliterating a tiny spot in the lower brain also depended on luck. He hit the precise spot on the first attempt and was himself unable to repeat his feat on the next several tries.

His discovery of sugar in the liver (portal) vein which was discussed earlier depended upon very high concentrations of sugar. His chemical test would not have picked up sugar in the concentrations usually present. But Bernard's method of killing his animals was to cut through the spinal cord, which produced a sudden massive outpouring of nervous stimuli. One result of this was that the liver poured out sugar at levels that Bernard's relatively crude test was able to detect.

Other examples of luck, chance, serendipity – whatever it is called – could be adduced, but the point should be made. Some have objected to the contention that chance figured heavily in Bernard's successes, the implication being that such an admission would somehow detract from Bernard's greatness. In truth the opposite is a more reasonable conclusion. Unexpected results are a consistent feature of biological experimentation, as Bernard rightly insisted. It is a mark of ability to notice them at all and a step toward genius to turn such events into new and fruitful hypotheses. To a large extent a judgment on serendipity depends on how it is defined. If it means only chance, Bernard has to be counted among the luckiest scientists in the history of biology. But Pasteur maintained that "chance only favours the prepared mind," and in this sense serendipity became just one more element in Bernard's mastery of the science of experimental medicine.

Technology and Specialization

Another meaning can be derived from the work of Claude Bernard. His era spanned the period during which the basic sciences and technology were becoming increasingly important in the struggle to understand the mechanisms of disease. The late development of biochemistry and its application to medicine has already been suggested in pointing out that the reagents available to Bernard would not detect blood sugar in normal concentrations. This situation changed drastically as the nineteenth century progressed. Chemistry and physics were now seen as necessary to the understanding of normal and pathological physiology. With this development came specialization, an eventuality Bernard himself saw when he said, "It is not possible to be an encyclopedist: one cannot demand that a man who is profound physiologist be at the same time a consummate chemist, physician, and mathematician."[9]

The movement gradually manifested itself in the educational process as well. Bernard was trained as a physician, as were the vast majority of medical scientists before him. As the twentieth century arrived, however, the split was well under way. Thereafter the trend would be toward specialized training for basic research, while the medical degree was used as preparation for medical practice, or for a few, clinical or bedside research.

Laboratory Medicine

One final extension of anatomical thinking in the cloak of physiology remains to be examined. It has been shown that the benefits of anatomical pathology for practicing physicians depended on improved tools of physical diagnosis. In analogous fashion the fruits of physiological pathology had to await the development of laboratory diagnosis. Bernard and the other physiologists of the nineteenth century were instrumental in bringing the laboratory to the bedside. When Bernard succeeded in determining one of the liver's functions by measuring what went in and out, he provided medicine with a model that had far-reaching potential. He was, in a word, studying the *function* of an organ. If normal function could be measured, then of course so could abnormal function.

The important impetus toward functional diagnosis occurred in Germany around 1867, when Adolf Kussmaul (1822–1902) decided that the stomach pump used in treating dilatation of the stomach might also be used for diagnostic purposes. The gastric contents, after all, must reflect the stomach's function. Kussmaul's lead was taken by Ottomar Rosenbach (1851–1907), who published a paper in 1878 which envisioned the broader aspects of studies under way on the function of the stomach. As a result of the application of steadily expanding biochemical understanding and improving technology, an entirely new dimension was added to the diagnosis of disease. The principal merit of laboratory medicine is its objectivity. Groups of diseases remained confused as long as physicians had to rely for diagnosis on nothing more than the patients' subjective accounts of their symptoms and the objective, but still relatively crude, findings of the physical examination. Many diseases were quickly separated from their mimes by the use of chemical tests and X rays. Simultaneously, the mechanisms by which diseases produce their deleterious effects gradually began to be understood, and with this came a rational basis for the prevention and cure of many diseases. For the most part these developments had to await the twentieth century, but at least one conceptual benefit from the improvements in laboratory medicine came in the last quarter of the nineteenth century with the establishment of the notion that specific diseases have specific causes. This occurred in the instance of contagious diseases, another concept with roots in the distant past. It was this development that led to the acceptance of the germ theory and control over some of mankind's most venerable and deadly diseases.

Notes

1. Galen. *On the Natural Faculties,* A. J. Brock, tr. London: William Heinemann, 1916, pp. 51-61.
2. Keynes, G. *The Life of William Harvey.* Oxford: Clarendon Press, 1966, p. 179.
3. Camac, C.N.B. *Classics of Medicine and Surgery.* New York: Dover Publications, 1959, p. 73.
4. Holmes, F. L. *Claude Bernard and Animal Chemistry.* Cambridge: Harvard University Press, 1974, pp. 437, 438, 440.
5. Henderson, L. J. Introduction to *An Introduction to the Study of Experimental Medicine,* by C. Bernard, trans. Henry Copley Greene. 1927. Reprint. New York: Dover Publications, 1957, p. vi.
6. Bernard, C. *Introduction à l'étude de la médicine expérimentale.* Paris: J. B. Baillière et Fils, 1865, pp. 267-268. My translation.
7. Lonsdale, K. "Origin of Serendipity," *Science* 142:621, 1963.
8. Bernard, *Introduction to Experimental Medicine.* P. 151.
9. Holmes, *Claude Bernard and Animal Chemistry.* P. 452.

Bibliographic Commentary

Happily for students of medicine in antiquity, translations of Galen continue to be made. For the purposes of this chapter, the most important existing translation is by A. J. Brock, Galen, *On the Natural Faculties,* London: William Heinemann, 1916. Important interpretive elements are found in O. Temkin, *Galenism: Rise and Decline of a Medical Philosophy,* Ithaca: Cornell University Press, 1973; J. Scarborough, *Roman Medicine,* London: Camelot Press, 1969; M. R. Cohen and I. E. Drabkin, *A Source Book in Greek Science,* New York: McGraw-Hill Book Co., 1948; and K. D. Keele, "Three Early Masters of Experimental Medicine – Erasistratus, Galen and Leonardo da Vinci," *Proc. Roy. Soc. Med.* 54:577–588, 1961.

Our current understanding of the motion of the blood in Galen's system is put forth by D. Fleming, "Galen on the Motions of the Blood in the Heart and Lungs," *Isis* 46:14–21, 1955. Attempts at dating Harvey's first conception of circulation are made by G. Keynes, *The Life of William Harvey,* Oxford: Clarendon Press, 1966, and more persuasively by J. J. Bylebyl, "The Growth of Harvey's *De Motu Cordis,*" *Bull. Hist. Med.* 47:427–470, 1973. These authors discuss the elusive elements that led to the idea that the blood circulates, a conundrum that occupies W. Pagel as well, in *William Harvey's Biological Ideas: Selected Aspects and Historical Background,* New York: Hafner, 1967, and H. Cohen in "The Germ of an Idea, or What Put Harvey on the Scent?" *J. Hist. Med. and Allied Sciences* 12:102–105, 1957. A fine overview of the entire climate in which Harvey made his discovery is found in J. J. Bylebyl, ed., *William Harvey and His Age: The Professional and Social Context of the Discovery of the Circulation of the Blood,* Baltimore: Johns Hopkins University Press, 1979. The importance of Harvey's method relative to his discovery itself has been explored by W. Pagel, *New Light on William Harvey,* Basel: S. Karger, 1976.

Examples of quantification in physiological experimentation before Harvey have been pointed out by R. H. Shryock, "The History of Quantification in Medical Science," *Isis* 52:215–237, 1961, and in two articles by O. Temkin, "Nutrition from Classical Antiquity to the Baroque," in *Human Nutrition, Historic and Scientific,* edited by I. Galdston, New York: International Universities Press, 1960, and "A Galenic Model for Quantitative Physiological Reasoning?" in *The Double Face of Janus,* Baltimore: Johns Hopkins University Press, 1977.

The best biography of Bernard is by J.M.D. Olmsted and E. H. Olmsted, *Claude Bernard and the Experimental Method in Medicine,* New York: Henry Schuman, 1952.

The 1970s saw a surge of interest in translating Bernard and assessing his accomplishments and method: C. Bernard, *Lectures on the Phenomena of Life Common to Animals and Plants,* vol. 1, translated by H. H. Hoff, R. Guillemin, and L. Guillemin, Springfield, Ill.: Charles C. Thomas, 1974; C. Bernard, *Claude Bernard's Revised Edition of His "Introduction à l'étude de la médicine expérimentale,"* edited by P. F. Cranefield, New York: Science History Publications, 1976; C. Bernard, *Notes pour le Rapport sur les progrès de la physiologie,* with comments by M. D. Grmek, Paris: Collège de France, 1979; and M. D. Grmek, *Raisonnement expérimental et recherches toxicologiques chez Claude Bernard,* Geneva: Librairie Droz, 1973. The source I have largely relied on in this section is F. L. Holmes, *Claude Bernard and Animal Chemistry,* Cambridge: Harvard University Press, 1974.

The concept of the *milieu intérieur* is discussed by the Olmsteds (p. 107) and in greater detail by Hoff and the Guillemins, (pp. 83–91). W. Cannon's extrapolation to include the concept of homeostasis is in W. Cannon, *The Wisdom of the Body,* New York: W. W. Norton & Company, 1932.

S. J. Reiser covers the importance of the basic sciences and technology in *Medi-*

cine and the Reign of Technology, Cambridge: Cambridge University Press, 1978. The development of the idea of functional disease and the rise of laboratory medicine are traced in the remarkable book by K. Faber, *Nosography in Modern Internal Medicine,* New York: Paul B. Hoeber, 1923.

Also of great utility is A. B. Davis, *Medicine and Technology,* Westport, Conn.: Greenwood Press, 1981.

8
SPECIFIC CAUSATION

It will be recalled that Morgagni titled his epochal publication *On the Seats and Causes of Disease.* In so doing he missed his mark by half. He succeeded in locating the seats of disease, but he was unable to do much with their causes. He did devote some effort to poisons as etiologic agents, but on the natural causes of disease he failed to shed much light. In part the difficulty related to an inherent limitation of the process of gross clinical-pathological correlation. As Osler put the matter, "Observation alone could give a complete knowledge *de sedibus,* but never *de causis morborum.*"[1] Morgagni is scarcely to be criticized in this regard. His book appeared in 1761; a century later, which is to say only 100 years ago, physicians did not know the cause of a single important human disease.

As it developed, specific etiology was first established in contagious diseases. This in itself is an interesting and little considered historical fact. Why contagious diseases? Why not an endocrine disease such as diabetes, or a malignant disease such as leukemia? For one thing the epidemic nature of contagious diseases — the sheer numbers involved — was bound to keep them in the forefront of lay and medical thinking. Five thousand deaths from smallpox in young people over a three-week period demand more attention than the same number of deaths among the aged spread over a year. For another, the nature of the contagious process itself provides a ready starting point for theorization and experimentation that is not found in other categories of disease. By definition contagious diseases spread from one person to another. This immediately raises questions. How does disease get from person to person? What is it that is being transmitted? Why the consistent pattern of spread in such diseases as smallpox and measles, and the erratic picture seen in cholera, plague, and yellow fever? Why do some persons in close contact with the sick escape unscathed and others with no apparent exposure fall ill and die? These questions arise quite naturally in contagious disease, but not in most other medical conditions.

The modern reader automatically associates contagion with germs. Historically this was not the case. The notion that contagious diseases were due to tiny living organisms recurred periodically over the centuries, but it was only one explanation among many. In fact, the concept was at one of its lowest ebbs during the decades immediately preceding the final ascendancy of the germ theory in the late nineteenth century.

The reader who ventures into the older literature may be confused by such terms as infection, contagion, and miasm. In their origin all three were thought of as pollutions, although contagions were held to operate principally by direct contact. By the sixteenth century a distinction had been made; infections could arise spontaneously and then, via the mechanism of contagion, could be passed on to a susceptible person. This notion persisted at least to around 1850, though by that time much confusion surrounded the terms. At times they were used synonymously. When differentiated, infections were thought to derive almost exclusively from emanations from decaying or diseased animals or other organized bodies, miasms as they were called. Contagions, on the other hand, were diseases which could not be attributed to any cause other than communication, either direct or indirect, with persons already suffering the disease. The confusion surrounding infection and contagion which endured in medical minds for some three hundred years began to dissipate as the germ theory developed in the last half of the nineteenth century.

Contagion Before the Nineteenth Century

It is a source of persistent mystery to historians that the ancient Greeks were all but "blind to the fact of contagion." According to most interpretations there is no reference whatever to contagion in the Hippocratic writers, and in fact contagion is scarcely mentioned in any classical medical literature. Nowhere do we find mention of measles, scarlet fever, or smallpox, all communicable diseases featuring highly visible and distinctive manifestations in the skin. The first systematic coverage of contagious diseases did not appear until the publication around A.D. 900 of an Arabic text, the *Book of Treasure.*

The idea of contagion became firmly entrenched in the Latin West with the acceptance of the Jewish Old Testament as a holy book in the Christian religion, particularly because of ideas concerning leprosy, which by then was prominent in medieval thinking. The arrival of bubonic plague, as mentioned earlier, unequivocally impressed the reality of contagion on the minds of all concerned. In a prescient passage in his treatise *On Plague,* the fourteenth-century Arabic physician Ibn al-Khatīb wrote, "The existence of contagion is established by experience, study, and the evidence of the senses, by trustworthy reports on transmission by garments, vessels, ear-rings; by the spread of it by persons from one house, by infection of a healthy sea-port by an arrival from an infected land."[2]

In this passage we find distinct intimations of the essential elements of the doctrine of contagion that would be elaborated two centuries later by the Renaissance physician Girolamo Fracastoro (1478–1553). As a result of his observations of plague and the new "French Disease" (syphilis), Fracastoro reformulated a theoretical basis for the spread of communicable diseases that offered practical measures for combating epidemics long before the advent of the germ theory. In his *De contagione* (1546) he outlined three routes by which contagious diseases spread: (1) direct person to person contact, as in syphilis, (2) spread by fomes, that is, inanimate objects such as bedclothing and eating utensils, and (3) infection from a distance, through miasms for example. Fracastoro's role in the development of the germ theory has been overstated at times, but what cannot be safely disputed is that his book was genuinely influential. *De contagione* remained the most authoritative single work on contagious diseases for some three hundred years.

Even though Fracastoro could not prove his theses by the standards of today's science, his observations and conclusions reaffirmed practical means for dealing with epidemic diseases. The sick could be isolated, their belongings burned, and quarantines established. How effective these measures were in practice cannot be determined, but at least physicians and rulers now had a rational course to follow.

Early Nineteenth-Century Anticontagionism

Having credited Fracastoro with helping to place contagionism on a sound theoretical footing in the sixteenth century, it becomes necessary to admit that the doctrine was again a matter of genuine dispute by the first half of the nineteenth century. The reasons for this turnabout can only be touched on here. In the seventeenth century Thomas Sydenham (baptized 1624, died 1689) led medical thinking away from contagionism by reviving the ancient concept of the epidemic constitution. In the Hippocratic writings, particularly in *Epidemics* and in *Airs, Waters, Places*, certain diseases were associated with particular seasons or climatic conditions. This general thesis was elaborated by Sydenham, although in a greatly revised form. In part, he said:

There are different constitutions in different years. They originate neither in their heat nor their cold, their wet nor their drought; but they depend upon certain hidden and inexplicable changes within the bowels of the earth. By the effluvia from these the atmosphere becomes contaminate, and the bodies of men are predisposed and determined, as the case may be, to this or that complaint. This continues during the influence of this or that constitution, which, after the cycle of a few years, gives ground, and makes way for another.[3]

Sydenham's lucid championing of this old idea was bound to influence those who followed. Rather than view his synthesis as erroneous theorization gone rampant, it is better to see the epidemic constitution as one example of a theory which explained, as well as any other at the time, certain observable facts of the epidemiology of contagious diseases.

The nature of the individual epidemic also shaped a given physician's philosophy of contagionism. Fracastoro became a contagionist in part due to his experience with syphilis. The celebrated American physician Benjamin Rush (1746-1813), on the other hand, shifted from contagionism to anticontagionism after his experience with the 1793 yellow fever epidemic in Philadelphia. The sporadic distribution of yellow fever by way of mosquito bites offered Rush none of the comforting consistency Fracastoro had detected in the venereal spread of syphilis.

The disputed state of contagionism in the first half of the nineteenth century is a near-perfect example of how the same evidence can be used by opposing parties to arrive at altogether discrepant conclusions. It can be a properly humbling story as well, because it demonstrates that even today an objective reading of the available evidence permits a defensible stand on either side of the issue. And finally, the battle over contagionism reveals that these matters are rarely decided on purely scientific grounds. It was not merely accident that so many leading anticontagionists were medical scientists, who, having recognized the tyranny of the dogma they had inherited, were determined to throw off the fetters of tradition, to examine everything anew, and to decide the issue on the basis of facts alone. Economic considerations also played a role. The discussion of contagionism was never limited to the medical evidence but always included the questionable value of quarantine. Here the anticontagionist ranks were joined by a rapidly expanding group of merchants and industrialists for whom quarantine meant loss of money, coupled with what was perceived as stifling bureaucratic domination.

This combination of liberal medical scientists (liberals generally opposed governmental intervention at this time), merchants, and industrialists finally held sway. In 1828 the French Academy of Medicine recommended effective repeal of the quarantine law of 1822. Because of the prestige of the academy, the move had a genuine impact, not only on quarantine practices, but on contagionism as a viable explanation of epidemic disease.

It should be emphasized that among physicians there were few absolute anticontagionists. Even the extremists acknowledged the contagiousness of measles, smallpox, gonorrhea, and syphilis. The argument raged mostly over the "big three," plague, yellow fever, and cholera. Here the evidence appeared to demand some measure of opposition to contagionism. Contagion as the spread of an agent directly from person to person or through the air for short distances simply did not square with observations everyone agreed to. Patients fell ill when no such influence existed, or remained unaffected while all around others succumbed. Epidemics arose apparently spontaneously, then for no apparent reason failed to spread beyond certain limits. Understanding of epidemics of yellow fever and cholera did not come even with the establishment of the germ theory itself, but only after the discovery that diseases could be spread by many intermediaries, in this case by germ-laden mosquitos and infected water supplies.

The epidemics of cholera that struck Britain and the United States had an important impact on the sanitary movement, as we shall see in the next chapter. But there was nothing in the often sporadic spread of cholera which could resolve the question of contagionism in any ultimate sense. During the outbreak of 1849, as with the earlier epidemic of 1832, most American physicians continued to find the cause of cholera in the atmosphere, although they were now trying to identify more precise etiologic agents, such as electricity, ozone, or carbonic acid. But the contagionists' case was soon to be reinforced, this time in a way that implicated medical attendants themselves in the spread of a particularly cruel disease, the nemesis of lying-in women in the nineteenth century, puerperal or childbed fever.

Semmelweis and Childbed Fever

Obstetrics is ordinarily the happiest of medical specialties. In the vast majority of cases the obstetrician is not even dealing with disease. Excepting disappointment over the sex of the new citizen, the "patient" is almost invariably satisfied with her obstetrical encounter. The mortality of childbirth has now been reduced to near zero, and the prospective mother can choose how little pain she wishes to bear. But the giving of birth was not always such a benign affair. In the nineteenth century the happiness accompanying an announcement of pregnancy was usually beclouded by a realistic fear. The morbidity and mortality associated with childbirth were a source of genuine concern to patients and physicians alike. The chief reason for this widespread anxiety was the often fatal complication, childbed fever.

When the placenta separates from the uterine wall after delivery of a child, a large wound remains, which has been likened to an amputation stump. Ordinarily this presents no danger because the uterus harbors no bacteria. But with the cervix widely dilated following the birth process, bacteria present in the vagina have access to the placental wound, and from there through the open veins and lymphatics to the bloodstream and the body at large. Normally the probability is small that pathogenic bacteria will be present in the vagina to ascend into the uterus after delivery. Any number of factors can enlarge this probability, but for our purposes the most important is the intrusion of a contaminated hand or instrument.

To get a clearer impression of the magnitude of the problem presented by puerperal fever in the nineteenth century, we return to Vienna, where we left Auenbrugger almost a hundred years earlier. There in the late eighteenth century the empress Maria Theresa, free for a while from the demands of war, turned her attention to the general well-being of her subjects. One manifestation of this monarchical altruism, one that was not finally accomplished until four years after her death, was the General Hospital of Vienna and its famous division, the Vienna Lying-in. At its dedication the Lying-in was the largest such institution in the world, a distinction that would have been a source of a good deal less pride if all concerned had known then what was seen in retrospect, that the total burden of postoperative and obstretrical infection was greater in hospitals than in homes and that the heaviest mortality was occurring in the larger hospitals.

The Vienna Lying-in was a teaching hospital, providing instruction to medical students and young physicians in its First Division, and after about 1840 or so, separate supervision of aspiring midwives in its Second Division. In order to keep track of the progress of labor, expectant mothers underwent periodic

pelvic examinations. The presence of students increased the incidence of such intrusions, at times several-fold. In the absence of
an established germ theory, physicians, nurses, and students engaged in handwashing largely for esthetic purposes, not with the
idea of preventing disease. Interspersed with their attendance on
women in labor, students and physicians were frequently involved in autopsies, many on women dead of puerperal fever. It
was in this setting on July 1, 1846, that a young Hungarian physician arrived to assume his duties as assistant at the First Obstetrical Clinic.

Ignaz Phillip Semmelweis (1818–1865) was born in a region
that is now located in Budapest. He began the study of law at the
University of Vienna but switched to medicine, receiving his
degree in April, 1844. In his position as assistant in obstetrics,
Semmelweis was soon confronted with a set of statistics that had
long disturbed medical attendants. Over the preceding years,
figures revealed that the mortality from childbed fever in the
First Division was some three times greater than in the Second.
In truth the figures were even worse than Semmelweis first realized, because seriously ill patients from the First Division were
frequently transferred to the General Hospital, where their
deaths were not recorded as puerperal fever. Such transfers
rarely occurred from the Second Division.

The discrepancy between the two divisions was so alarming
that even the laity of Vienna knew it well. As Semmelweis later
wrote,

That they were afraid of the First Division there was abundant evidence.
Many heartrending scenes occurred when patients found out that they
had entered the First Division by mistake. They knelt down, wrung
their hands and begged that they might be discharged. Lying-in patients
with uncountable pulse, meteoric (swollen) abdomen, and dry tongue,
only a few hours before their death, would protest that they were really
quite well, in order to avoid medical treatment, for they believed that
the doctor's interference was always the precursor of death.

The psychological impact of such a situation is difficult, perhaps impossible, to grasp in our era of benign childbirth. The
chapel of the lying-in hospital was so located that the priestly
procession involved in last rites had to pass through five wards
of the First Division to reach the sickroom. Ordinarily this ritual

was observed only once daily, but the death rate from puerperal fever was such that the priests at times were recalled soon after their scheduled visit. Again in Semmelweis's words: "Even to me myself it had a strange effect upon my nerves when I heard the bell hurried past my door; a sigh would escape my heart for the victim that once more was claimed by an unknown power. The bell was a painful exhortation to me to search for this unknown cause with all my might."

For a year Semmelweis accumulated data and struggled to make sense of the facts confronting him. Why were women who were admitted after giving birth on the way to the hospital (*Gassengeburt*, or streetbirths, they were called) rarely affected by puerperal fever? Why had the death rate jumped suddenly from 0.84 percent in 1821 to 7.8 percent in 1822, the year following Doctor Klein's appointment to the chair of obstetrics? And why the appalling difference between the medical student and midwife wards in the first place? "Everywhere questions arose," he wrote; "everything remained without explanation: all was doubt and difficulty. Only the great number of the dead was an undoubted reality."

Depressed by such questions and by political considerations that forced him to repeat his two-year period as ordinary assistant, Semmelweis left for Venice to freshen his spirits. Soon after his return he learned of the death of Professor Kolletschka who, in the course of a post-mortem had suffered a scalpel wound at the hands of one of his students. From the autopsy protocol Semmelweis learned that Kolletschka had been "affected with lymphangitis, phlebitis in the same upper extremity, and he died from pleurisy, pericarditis, peritonitis, and meningitis, and a few days before his death metastasis occurred in one of the eyes." Reading this, Semmelweis's thinking took a crucial leap.

In the excited condition in which I then was, it rushed into my mind with irresistible clearness that the disease from which Kolletschka had died was identical to that from which I had seen so many hundreds of lying-in women die. [They] also died from phlebitis, lymphangitis, peritonitis, pleuritis, meningitis, and in them also metastases sometimes occurred. Day and night the vision of Kolletschka's malady haunted me, and with ever increasing conviction I recognised the identity of the disease from which Kolletschka died with the malady which I had observed to carry off so many lying-in women.[4]

With this, the puzzling pieces fell into place. Kolletschka, though a man, had in effect died of childbed fever. In his case the disease was transmitted from the dead body to his bloodstream by a scalpel wound. In the case of childbed fever the disease was carried unwittingly on the hands of medical attendants from women sick or dead of puerperal fever to normal lying-in women. The women who gave birth on the way to the hospital were spared childbed fever because they avoided the pelvic examinations that spread the disease.

Also comprehensible was the sudden jump in the incidence of puerperal fever in 1822, when Klein took over the obstetrical unit. Klein's predecessor had refused to accede to demands from his superiors that the various aspects of labor be taught directly from cadavers. Instead he had insisted on using manikins of the pelvis and child, or phantoms as they were called. Under administrative pressure, when Klein took over he agreed to use fresh cadavers for instructing midwives as well as medical students. Many of the cadavers, of course, had reached their tragic end as a result of puerperal fever, and were thus a rich source of infective material easily transmissible from the classroom sessions involving dead bodies to women in labor on the wards. Similarly clear were the statistics that had first attracted Semmelweis's attention. Medical personnel in the First Division were customarily involved in autopsies, an infrequent situation in the Second Division for either teachers or pupils.

Perhaps no disease in history has matched puerperal fever in demonstrating the role that medical ignorance, understandable though it may be, can play in binding the physician directly to his patient's death. Practices such as bloodletting at times undoubtedly abetted the disease instead of recovery, but precision is elusive here because the medical intervention cannot be separated from the natural course of the disease. In the case of puerperal fever the relationship between the medical attendants and the deaths of their patients was now starkly visible. The confessions of physicians, before and after Semmelweis, who were gradually moved to conclude that they had been agents in the spread of childbed fever, makes for some of the most poignant reading in the annals of disease.

Convinced of the mechanism by which puerperal fever was

being spread, Semmelweis now faced the problem of remedying the situation. He had concluded that the agents responsible for childbed fever were cadaveric particles, that is, morbific or dead materials, passed from the sick and dead to healthy women on the hands of medical attendants. Finding that he could not remove the odor of this morbific matter with soap and water, he reasoned that some of the particles must survive even a thorough washing. In order to destroy the odor, which he equated with the morbific material, he decided first on a chlorine solution, switching later to the cheaper chlorinated lime. Before moving from the autopsy room to a woman in labor or from one patient to another, all medical attendants were required to undergo a chlorine rinse.

The efficacy of Semmelweis's method was soon apparent. In 1846, before chlorine was adopted, the mortality rate was 2.7 percent in the Second Division and 11.4 percent in the First Division. In 1848, after a full year of the chlorine wash, for the first time in the history of the Vienna Lying-in, the mortality rate in the First Division was lower than in the Second, 1.27 percent versus 1.33 percent.

The rest of Semmelweis's story need only be touched on here. One author spoke of the "annihilating force" of Semmelweis's statistics, but instead of enjoying an easy victory, the Immortal Magyar became involved in disputes that lasted until his death in 1865. His initial results were published in December, 1847. A decade later Semmelweis's doctrine was thoroughly discredited in Germany and France, although it fared somewhat better in Great Britain, particularly in Scotland. The reasons for this slow acceptance are complex and numerous. The revolution of 1848 distracted attention from his discovery and left Semmelweis on the losing political side when order was finally restored. Repeatedly, because of his personality, he failed to capitalize on chances to propound the merits of his convictions. He was averse to scientific writing, so that publicity for his doctrine depended on letters sent around Europe by his supporters. A fully developed account of his method and results did not appear until he published *Kindbettfiebers* in 1861.

Further, there was the situation within the medical profession. We have already seen that the whole question of contagionism was being disputed at the time. Beyond that, and impossible to assess with any hope of accuracy, is the awful psychological burden inherent in accepting Semmelweis's doctrine. It is easy to accuse his opposition of culpable negligence, but one need not ponder the matter long to agree that physicians were being asked to accept an almost unbearable load of guilt, and all on the basis of a few statistics which, in any event, carried nothing like the weight they would have in our day. Given the circumstances, perhaps the most implausible scenario one might imagine for the years immediately after Semmelweis's first announcement would have been a general and ready acceptance of his novel and threatening revelations.

So it was that years later directors of maternity hospitals were still puzzling over epidemics of childbed fever. In 1864 in the Paris Maternity Hospital, 310 deaths occurred among 1,350 confinements, and the hospital had to be closed the next year. Indeed, as it turned out, things were not as simple as Semmelweis or his supporters believed. The microbes of puerperal fever are ubiquitous and not limited to the hands of medical personnel. They can be found normally on the skin of lying-in women, in hospital bedclothing, in droplets spread by coughing and sneezing, and in many other places. An antiseptic handwash was only a partial solution, as Semmelweis himself discovered when he was unable to duplicate his Vienna success after returning to his native Budapest.

With the mode of infection generally understood in our era of asepsis and antibiotics, it might be supposed that puerperal fever is now of interest only to medical historians. It is a measure of the complexity of the situation to find that such is not the case. In 1965 at the Boston Hospital for Women (Lying-in Division), for the first time in thirty-three years an epidemic of puerperal fever broke out. Before it was brought under control eleven days later, 20 of the 137 women delivered during that period exhibited the clinical picture of puerperal fever, and 16 had positive cultures to the same type of streptococcus. Current obstetrical texts still indict physicians as frequent vehicles in the spread of the disease. And so it apparently turned out in the Boston episode. Sophisticated epidemiological detective work concluded that the most probable focus of infection was an anesthetist who harbored the organisms under two scabs, on wounds so tiny he had not even noticed them. The professional stigmata associated with childbed fever also remain. An article written in 1934 told of a survey of twenty-nine outbreaks of puerperal fever, yet only one hospital had the "scientific candor" to report its experiences in the medical literature.

With his book of 1861 Semmelweis did not establish the doctrine of contagionism. Indeed, it is an indicator of the prevailing confusion that he himself did not believe puerperal fever was contagious in the sense that the disease could spread directly from one woman to another. Rather, he perceived it more in the nature of an infection, which presupposed the intervention of some intermediate agent, in this case the morbific or cadaveric particles from the dead or dying. In the mid-nineteenth century all manner of evidence had been accumulated suggesting that certain diseases were contagious. Yet another mass of data existed that simply would not square with contagionism. At this point the situation was reminiscent of the problem of the etiology of cancer today. What was missing was a new approach, a new experiment that would reconcile the apparently contradictory evidence. Semmelweis concluded that something was being transferred from woman to woman on the hands of medical attendants, but what was its nature? Later work would show that it was not the dead particles he suspected, but the selfsame tiny animals which had appeared and reappeared many times in the history of disease.

The Animalcular Theory

The notion that invisible animals might be responsible for contagious disease has been variously called the animalcular theory and the doctrine of *contagium animatum* or *contagium vivum*. As early as 1557 Jerome Cardan (1501-1576) suggested that the seeds of disease might be living and reproducing. The Jesuit priest Athanasius Kircher (1602?-1680) is credited with the first explicit statement on *contagium animatum*. It is all but certain that Kircher did not see the causative bacteria in the blood of plague victims, as he claimed, but he can at least be credited with the idea of using the microscope to search for tiny animals in disease. The Dutch microscopist Antoni Van Leeuwenhoek (1632–1723) unquestionably found bacteria in scrapings from his own teeth in 1674. His microscope, like Kircher's, should not have permitted Leeuwenhoek to see creatures as small as those we know from his drawings he was able to see. He admits he kept some special technique a secret, but despite conjecture, no one has been able to resolve the mystery.

In the eighteenth century it is possible to find remarkably accurate conclusions on the role of little animals in disease, but all these conclusions suffered the same failing that accounted for the ebbs and flows of contagionism generally; they remained immune to convincing proof. Leeuwenhoek's findings, for example, could be turned around to serve admirably the cause of the anticontagionists. If, after all, he had hundreds of such creatures in his mouth at any given moment and simultaneously enjoyed good health, what more was needed to prove that bacteria do not cause disease?

The nineteenth century saw an increase in experimentation, including the use of the microscope. From this effort, isolated discoveries emerged which favored the animalcular theory. For most scientists of the time, however, the case remained unpersuasive. Justus von Liebig (1803–1873), a towering figure in chemistry at the time, echoed the thinking of many scientists on the animalcular question when he wrote in 1845, "As to the opinion which explains putrefaction of animal substances by the presence of microscopic animalculae, it may be compared to that of a child who would explain the rapidity of the Rhine current by attributing it to the violent movement of the numerous mill wheels of Mayence."[5] In short, the animalcular theory was nothing more than a childish illusion.

Not surprisingly, then, we arrive at the mid-nineteenth century with the animalcular theory involved in the same dispute as contagionism generally. The two were part and parcel, and indeed the existence of a *contagium animatum* placed a greater tax on credulity than contagionism alone, which at least had the analogy of chemical poisoning to fall back on. The denouement, as it turned out, would not be based on a direct revelation that microbial organisms cause human disease but on the discovery that they cause fermentations, and that each fermentation springs from its own specific microorganism.

Fermentation, Putrefaction, and Wound Infection

The question of whether the microorganisms that were consistently associated with fermentative reactions were responsible for the observed chemical transformation engaged some of the best scientific minds of the nineteenth century. The obvious problem was that the living organisms could as easily be the result as the cause of a given fermentation, or even a coincidental occurrence, and thus of no importance to either side of the question. The individual who finally convinced the scientific world that fermentations depended on specific microbes was Louis Pasteur (1822–1895). The ramifications of his proof, in his hands and others, would run beyond the obvious implications for industrial chemistry and speak directly to the concept of specific causation in human disease.

Pasteur was born in Dôle in eastern France in 1822 and was educated as a chemist. We encounter him in the 1850s at a time before it became unfashionable for academic scientists to be involved in the mundane application of their talents. Pasteur, in the process of assisting a merchant to overcome difficulties he was having with the alcoholic fermentation of beet sugar, became interested in the problem of fermentations generally. Fermentation at the time meant the apparently spontaneous transformation in organic substances that produced such chemicals as alcohol and acetic acid. The term was loosely dissociated from the process of putrefaction by which meat, eggs, and other natural substances spoiled.

The core question of fermentation and putrefaction was whether these phenomena were purely chemical or due to living organisms. Pasteur leaned toward a biological etiology, and in this he had a long line of precursors. As far back as the Talmud a remarkable comparison had appeared between reproduction and fermentation, and from then on each epoch had its champions of the biochemical view. This long and complex story cannot be explored here; rather it can only be asserted that before Pasteur the matter had been long disputed, with neither side able to provide definitive proof.

In a series of experiments between 1860 and 1870, Pasteur not only proved that microorganisms were responsible for fermentations, but demonstrated that each fermentation was the product of a specific microorganism. Further, he showed that the germs that caused fermentations were ubiquitous, existing even on dust particles in the air.

This phase of Pasteur's work was soon applied to sick human beings, but not, as it developed, by the French chemist himself. Sometime around 1865 a professor of surgery at Glasgow University, the Englishman Joseph Lister (1827-1912), learned of Pasteur's work. Was it not possible, Lister reasoned, that putrefaction in wounds might have the same cause as fermentations, that is, germs falling into the wound from the air? If so, there was the possibility at least of taking some sort of preventive measure.

The problem of wound infection before antisepsis is among those which cannot be imagined today. Postoperative infection was so firmly associated with hospitals that the term "hospitalism" was coined to describe the role played by houses of healing in fostering wound infections. As early as 1801 John Bell (1763-1820) called attention to the phenomenon, saying that the only hope for patients with gangrene was to get them out of the hospital, to "hurry them out of this house of death," to "lay them in a schoolroom, a church, on a dunghill, or in a stable," to "carry them anywhere but to their graves."[6] The presence of infected wounds was so constant that it had been believed for centuries that pus was necessary for healing; "laudable pus" it came to be called.

Lister decided to test his elaboration of Pasteur's experimental findings by applying them to the treatment of compound fractures, breaks in which the bone has penetrated the skin. Because such wounds almost invariably became infected, union of the bones often failed to occur. Gangrene and amputation followed, and mortality was discouragingly high. If contaminating germs were responsible for the infection and could be killed or kept from the wound, presumably a compound fracture could be managed as successfully as a simple one.

According to his story, Lister seized on carbolic acid as an antiseptic agent after reading an account describing the chemical's use in purifying sewage and in the treatment of certain animal parasites in cattle. If so, he was ignorant of the fact that the chemical had been used for years for its healing and antiseptic purposes. Just two years before Lister adopted it, carbolic acid had been advocated for use in all manner of disease by the Frenchman François Jules Lemaire (1814–1886).

In 1865 Lister began applying carbolic acid antisepsis to cases of compound fracture. A piece of cloth was soaked in crude carbolic acid and inserted into the wound. Over this a carbolic acid dressing was applied, followed by a thin piece of tin or lead to hinder evaporation. The first patient died, as Lister admitted, "of improper management." Of the next ten, nine survived, although one unfortunate had to undergo amputation. The significance of these figures can be measured against Lister's own experience with amputations, wherein the mortality rate was 45 percent in the period 1864–1866. One of his early cases involved a compound fracture of the leg associated with soft tissue damage and hemorrhage into the muscle, ordinarily an ideal breeding ground for bacteria. In the words he wrote to his father, Lister's excitement can be detected even if buried in typical understatement.

Though hardly expecting success, I tried the application of carbolic acid to the wound to prevent decomposition of the blood, and so avoid the fearful mischief of suppuration throughout the limb. Well, it is now eight days since the accident, and the patient has been going on exactly as if there was no external wound, that is, as if the fracture were a simple one.[7]

Lister published his results in the *Lancet* in 1867 under the title "On a new Method of treating compound fractures, abscesses, etc." Under Pasteur's influence he first believed that germs entered wounds only through the air. This led him to adopt a method of spraying the entire operating room. He abandoned the method in 1887, but only after several years' experience had shown that airborne contamination was nothing compared to infection from clothing and the skin of the patient and the patient's attendants.

If Lister's method had been widely and immediately accepted, it would have implied tacit acceptance by the medical profession of the germ theory of disease. Once again the intellectual climate militated against such an easy victory. The doctrine spread gradually to the Continent, where it was welcomed, particularly in Germany. Still, many remained unconvinced, as indicated by the following account describing an episode in 1878.

One day, at the Hôtel Dieu, Professor Richet was asked by Pasteur to collect pus from one of the surgical cases. He was doing his ward rounds with a soiled white apron over his black dress suit. Interrupting himself, he said, "We are going to open this abscess; bring me the small alcohol lamp which M. Pasteur used yesterday to flame the tube in which he collected some pus for his experiment. We shall now sacrifice to the new fashion and flame the scalpel," and with a wide gesture, which was characteristic of him, he wiped the scalpel on the soiled apron twice, and then attacked the abscess.[8]

Clearly Pasteur's work on ferments and Lister's practical extension thereof would not be enough to establish that specific contagious diseases also had specific living causative agents. Before the main issue could be joined, Pasteur knew that the age-old doctrine of spontaneous generation would have to be laid to rest, and to that end he next applied the full talents of his experimental genius.

Pasteur and Contagion

Simply put, the doctrine of spontaneous generation holds that living organisms can arise spontaneously from matter independently of parents. At various times and for differing reasons the doctrine was generally accepted, even by reputable scientists employing the crudest of proofs. Johannes Helmont (1579-1644), the seventeenth-century chemist, who should not be judged by this one episode, gave a recipe for creating a mouse which could easily be tested by any doubter; one need only put some dirty linen in a box, add a few grains of wheat or a piece of cheese, and wait an appropriate length of time. Over ensuing centuries, most scientists rejected the possibility of spontaneous generation for larger animals but retained the theory to explain such phenomena as the appearance of maggots in rotting flesh.

Despite the fact that he failed to construct an experiment that proved spontaneous generation could not occur, Pasteur emerged triumphant in the controversy over spontaneous generation. It is now clear that he prevailed not only because of his scientific proofs, but for a variety of political and religious reasons as well. What matters here is not that he was unable to devise the definitive experiment but that he appeared to have done so.

He was now free to turn his full attention to the question of contagion proper.

At this point Pasteur had established at least three important tenets: he had demonstrated that fermentations depend on specific microorganisms; he had discredited spontaneous generation and in the process had equated fermentation with putrefaction; and in his work with silkworm disease, he had confirmed the finding that one kind of animal, in this case a type of protozoan, could produce disease in another kind of animal. As early as 1859 Pasteur was thinking about contagious diseases, but his interests were diluted by the demands of French industry. Gradually, however, the germ theory of disease became his driving ambition. By 1876 he was convinced that the microorganisms responsible for the "diseases" of wines and beer must have their counterparts among humans. In the end, however, the honor for making that connection would go to another.

Robert Koch

By 1876 or so a causal association between microorganisms and certain diseases was widely suspected. The questions were: Are human diseases involved? If so, which diseases are due to germs? and finally, How can the relationship be proved? By this time powerful achromatic microscopes were available, and selective staining of vital tissues was a promising new field, following the demonstration in 1875 that methyl violet would stain certain bacteria (cocci) in tissues. The difficulties in seeing tiny unstained microorganisms against a background that offers little contrast can be appreciated only by making the attempt. So it was that Robert Koch (1843–1910) had not only a more congenial ideological climate in which to pursue the germ theory, but a rapidly improving technology as well.

At the time he made his first important discovery, Koch was a practitioner in a community of some 4,000 persons in Wollstein, East Prussia. Unlike most American practitioners at the time, Koch had a sound scientific and experimental background, including training under the histologist Jakob Henle (1809–1885). In his daily rounds Koch had ample opportunity to observe splenic fever, or anthrax, a disease of serious import to domesticated animals in the area. As he took up the study of the disease, Koch learned that at least three investigators before him, P.-F.O. Rayer (1793-1867) and C. J. Davaine (1812-1882) in 1845 and F.A.A. Pollender (1800-1879) a decade later, had seen large numbers of rod-like bacteria in the blood of animals dead of anthrax. Pollender (and Davaine later) was convinced these bacteria could be the cause of the disease, but he soon encountered the inconsistency which had defeated all the best efforts before Koch—some animals injected with anthrax blood died without showing the rods in their blood. Even after Davaine returned to the problem with renewed vigor, those who tried to duplicate his efforts encountered the same inconsistency, plus another: some believed that they had succeeded in transmitting anthrax using blood that did not contain the rods. Despite the loopholes in Davaine's experimental results, both Koch and Pasteur would later recognize his work as the "first, unquestionable proof" of *contagium vivum.*

Koch unraveled the mystery by determining for the first time the complete life cycle of the anthrax organism. Using crude, homemade technology, he fashioned a warm-stage microscope which allowed him to keep the anthrax bacillus alive for long periods of time in an uncontaminated medium of serum or the aqueous humor from bullock eyes. He determined that the rod form of anthrax formed spores in the process of reproduction and that these spores, in contrast with the delicate rods, were highly resistant to destruction, even outside the body. Koch immediately seized on the importance of this finding. The rod stage produced the disease, and the spore stage was a reproductive phase which, if introduced into an animal, could again become a pathogenic rod. The inconsistency that had plagued Koch's predecessors was thus explained. Whether or not the blood from infected animals would infect other animals depended on whether it contained rods or spores. It all depended on the stage at which the blood was drawn. By judicious timing of the reproductive cycle, Koch was able to transfer anthrax bacilli from slide to slide through eight generations, each of which produced anthrax in experimental animals.

In his solution to the anthrax problem in 1876, Koch achieved a number of goals which were fundamental to the rapid development of bacteriology that followed. He delineated the complete life cycle of a pathogenic microorganism and demonstrated the critical value of such understanding. He cultivated what for practical purposes was a microbial pure culture outside a living animal, and he used that organism, free of other bacteria, to reproduce the disease in healthy animals at will. In terms of this chapter, specific causation had now been proved. The value of Koch's work was recognized immediately when he demonstrated it to one of the leading botanists of the time, Ferdinand Cohn (1828–1898). But anthrax was largely a disease of animals. Final proof for the germ theory in human beings would come six years later in 1882, when Koch announced that he had discovered the bacterial cause of tuberculosis, one of the most devastating of nineteenth-century contagions.

Here again Koch had shoulders to stand on. In 1868 a French army surgeon, Jean Antoine Villemin (1827–1892), had published a book entitled *Études sur la tuberculose* (Studies of Tuberculosis), wherein he described his success in transmitting tuberculosis from human beings to a variety of animals. This proved the contagiousness of consumption, but left him at the same impasse confronted by Semmelweis: What exactly was being transmitted? In 1882, using methylene blue as a stain, Koch announced that he had consistently identified the causative bacterium of tuberculosis in a wide variety of tissues. As with anthrax, he cultivated tuberculosis artificially and produced the characteristic lesions in guinea pigs, from which the organism could then be recovered. His accomplishment is all the more remarkable because, among human pathogens, the tubercle bacillus is one of the more difficult to stain and culture.

Koch's success with tuberculosis brought a host of scientists to the new field of bacteriology, and with them, the problems that usually accompany a major scientific discovery. The chief technical difficulty facing practitioners of the new science of bacteriology was that of obtaining a pure culture. Bacteria were grown in liquid broths at the time. If Leeuwenhoek had placed a scraping from his teeth in a liquid medium, he would have obtained a wild profusion of many different colonies from which a pure growth could not have been extracted. In an attempt to solve this difficulty, Pasteur had employed serial dilutions and may even have obtained pure cultures, but not in a way that permitted them to be grown consistently outside the animal's blood stream. Koch, perhaps drawing on the experience of others, devised a solid medium consisting of gelatin and meat extract. By dipping a sterile platinum ring into a broth culture and streaking it across his gelatin he spread out the individual bacteria, whereupon each formed its own pure colony. These were then transferred to tubes containing gelatin in a slanted position and allowed to grow further. For such a seemingly simple invention, Koch's solid medium produced remarkable results. The method was announced in 1881 at the International Medical Congress held in London, and immediately after the demonstration, according to Lister, Pasteur said to Koch, whom he had not met previously, "C'est un grand progrès, Monsieur."

The second great problem immediately facing the new bacteriologists was one of causality. The fact that a bacterium is found in conjunction with a given disease, even consistently, does not mean the two are causally related. In the seventeenth century, after Kircher announced his plague organisms, a number of writers "were seized with a sort of vermicular obsession," seeing worms everywhere, both in health and disease. During the 1870s and 1880s, fanciers of bacteriology fell under a similar spell of "ruthless and uncritical enthusiasm." Even Virchow, a bacterial doubter in his early years, erroneously adopted some of the many spurious causative agents emerging annually, smallpox bacteria, for instance, and a bacillus of beriberi.

Koch's teacher, Jakob Henle, had anticipated the problem by some thirty years. In a work entitled *Von den Miasmen und Kontagien* (On Miasmata and Contagions) published in 1840, he reasoned that before a germ could be held responsible for a disease it must be constantly associated with that disease. As refined by Koch in 1882 and 1890, the postulates required that:

1. The parasite occurs in every case of the disease in question and under circumstances which can account for the pathological changes and clinical course of the disease.

2. It occurs in no other disease as a fortuitous and nonpathogenic parasite.

3. After being fully isolated from the body and repeatedly grown in pure culture, it can induce the disease anew.[9]

In reality the elements of Koch's postulates had been fulfilled as early as 1841 by David Gruby (1810–1898), when he used potato slices to culture the trichophyton that causes favus, a fungus disease that centers largely on the human scalp. Gruby's work went largely unnoticed, in part because his poor clinical descriptions led to confusion over just what diseases his fungi caused. We now realize that the Henle-Koch postulates could not be applied rigidly to all the discoveries in microbiology that came along, but they did serve as a useful logical restraint during a particularly confusing period in the story of specific etiology.

Aftermath

By 1878 the concept of specific causation had spread even to nonmedical scientists. In that year the British physicist John Tyndall (1820–1893) was quoted as saying that "As surely as a thistle grows from a thistle seed, as surely as a fig comes from the fig, the grape from the grape, the thorn from the thorn, so surely does the typhoid fever virus increase and multiply into typhoid fever, the scarlatina virus into scarlet fever, the smallpox virus into smallpox."[10]

Tyndall was correct but a bit premature, because by 1881 only two diseases were known to have probable or certain bacterial causes, anthrax, as we have seen, and relapsing fever, in which an organism called a spirochete had been consistently demonstrated. After Koch identified the tubercle bacillus in 1882, the floodgates of bacterial discovery burst open. Before the end of the century microbial agents had been correctly associated with cholera, glanders, diphtheria, typhoid, gonorrhea, pneumococcal pneumonia, Malta fever, meningococcal meningitis, tetanus, plague, botulism, acute dysentery, and the numerous infections due to staphylococci and streptococci. By 1900 the germ theory was indisputably established. In the United States, where the practice of medicine remained largely derivative of that of Europe and nationalism was still a problem, acceptance was slow and spotty. But even here, in part because of the obvious advantages of Lister's antiseptic method, surgeons were embracing the germ theory in increasing numbers as the twentieth century arrived. It remains to ask two questions: To what extent did the germ theory as it existed in 1885 explain the observed facts of contagion? and What effect did the application of the theory have on human mortality and morbidity? The second of these will be reserved for a later treatment.

Discovery might be likened to the puzzle box in which each solution reveals a new problem. The work of Pasteur and Koch by no means accounted for all the phenomena observable in contagious diseases at the time. When he turned his attention to rabies, Pasteur unwittingly took up the study of a viral disease. Lacking the electron microscope, he was unable to see the organism, nor could he grow it on artificial media. Yet he could pass the disease serially from animal to animal. Thus immediately a contagious disease was encountered for which, as originally formulated, the Henle-Koch postulates were inadequate, a situation that recurred periodically as new knowledge developed. Pasteur was not deterred by such logical devices, however useful they might be in restraining less disciplined minds. He went on to develop a rabies vaccine without ever seeing the responsible virus or growing it outside its animal hosts.

The simplistic interpretation of the germ theory, one which many physicians embraced at first, was that a pathogenic bacterium in a human host equalled a disease. Before long it became clear that some individuals could harbor large numbers of dangerous bacteria and suffer no effects. The most famous of these was Mary Mallon, whose gallbladder teemed with typhoid bacilli while she enjoyed ordinary health. Typhoid Mary, as she came to be called, was employed as a cook in at least six different families between 1901 and 1907. Everywhere that Mary went, typhoid was sure to go. One estimate had her responsible for over two hundred cases and three deaths in the vicinity of New York City alone. Finally at the behest of the New York City Health Department she was hospitalized, found to be a typhoid carrier, and required to change her occupation. Mary escaped surveillance in 1910, then surfaced again as the likely cause of a typhoid outbreak involving some twenty-five cases at the Sloane Hospital for Women in New York. This time she was incarcerated until she died in 1938. A later investigation revealed that she had infected many other persons and may have been the locus of the typhoid epidemic in 1903, in which more than thirteen hundred persons were stricken. The carrier state is now recognized as extremely common in many diseases. Hospital personnel who harbor bacteria that have become resistant to antibiotics constitute an instructive and dangerous current variant of the phenomenon.

Next was the matter of host resistance. In 1878 Pasteur demonstrated the fact that alterations in an animal's physiology could determine its susceptibility to bacterial exposure. He demonstrated that under ordinary circumstances a hen could not be infected by anthrax. Knowing that hens had a higher body temperature than animals normally susceptible to the disease, he lowered the hens' temperature and found that he could infect them with anthrax as easily as other susceptible animals. The complexity of host resistance was dramatized by Max von Pettenkofer (1818–1901), a Munich hygienist, in 1892 when he deliberately swallowed one cubic centimeter of a culture of cholera bacilli diluted in water. For a gesture that might have killed certain susceptibles, Pettenkofer suffered nothing more than a "light diarrhea." Whether illness results from a given bacterial exposure is now seen to depend on many variables, including age, weight, sex, nutritional state, race, previous exposures, and genetic endowment as expressed in the individual's immune system. "In infective diseases attention must be directed to the soil as well as the seed."[11]

Nor did the work of Pasteur and Koch illuminate the inconsistency in disease spread that had forced Fracastoro to resort to miasms and rendered so puzzling the epidemics of plague, yellow fever, malaria, and other insect vector diseases throughout history. Here, it would be discovered, disease did not depend upon direct exposure or touching fomites, but upon an accidental encounter with a mosquito, tick, flea, or louse.

Even where insects were not involved, at times the mode of spread had to be uncovered before the epidemiological picture made sense. Cholera usually results from ingesting infected water or milk. Such is not the case with anthrax, where a break in the skin or mucous membrane is ordinarily required. Each infectious disease has its own mode of spread, some undergoing complicated life cycles involving several intermediate hosts. All of this remained obscure in the period immediately after the accomplishments of Koch and Pasteur.

The germ theory, then, did not turn out to be a final and fully formed synthesis. Just as with the Henle-Koch postulates, it required many amendments and modifications, a process that continues yet today. But even if the story had ended with Pasteur and Koch, it would have established another landmark in the conceptual history of disease – specific diseases have specific causes. Further, the bacteriologists of the late nineteenth century provided a rational basis for a number of attempts that were already under way to prevent human diseases, attempts which had been more or less successful but for reasons that were not well understood. Specificity in prevention, as we see next, was bound to improve with the demonstration that specific diseases have specific contagious causes.

Notes

1. Osler, W. "The Pathological Institute of a General Hospital," *Glasgow Med. J.* 76:324, 1911.

2. Arnold, T., and Guillaume, A. *The Legacy of Islam.* London: Oxford University Press, 1931, p. 340.

3. Latham, R. G., trans. *The Works of Thomas Sydenham.* London: The Sydenham Society, 1848, vol. 1, pp. 33-34.

4. The Semmelweis quotes are from Sinclair, W. J. *Semmelweis: His Life and His Doctrine.* Manchester: University Press, 1909, pp. 35-49.

5. Quoted in Vallery-Radot, R. *The Life of Pasteur.* New York: Doubleday, Page & Company, 1916, p. 175.

6. Bell, J. *Principles of Surgery.* Edinburgh: T. Cadell & W. Davies, 1801, vol. 1, p. 177.

7. Guthrie, D. *Lord Lister.* Baltimore: Williams and Wilkins Company, 1949, p. 60.

8. Dubos, R. *Louis Pasteur: Free Lance of Science.* Boston: Little, Brown & Company, 1950, p. 302.

9. Evans, A. S. "Causation and Disease: The Henle-Koch Postulates Revisited," *Yale J. Biol. and Med.* 49:177, 1976.

10. *Scientific American* 238:14, June 1978.

11. Rolleston, H. "Changes in the Character of Diseases," *Brit. Med. J.* 1:499, 1933.

Bibliographic Commentary

The contagious diseases have received more historical attention than any other group of human ailments. A number of general and specific works in this regard are listed in the bibliographic commentary for Chapter 2. Others include W.

Bulloch, *The History of Bacteriology*, London: Oxford University Press, 1938; W. W. Ford, *Bacteriology*, New York: Paul B. Hoeber, 1939; H. A. Lechevalier and M. Solotorovsky, *Three Centuries of Microbiology*, New York: McGraw-Hill Book Company, 1965; and R. H. Shryock, "Germ Theories in Medicine Prior to 1870: Further Comments on Continuity in Science," *Clio Medica* 7:81-109, 1972.

The distinctions made between infection and contagion follow O. Temkin, "An Historical Analysis of the Concept of Infection," in *The Double Face of Janus and Other Essays in the History of Medicine*, Baltimore: Johns Hopkins University Press, 1977. The revisionist view of Fracastoro has been presented convincingly by N. Howard-Jones, "Fracastoro and Henle: A Re-appraisal of their Contribution to the Concept of Communicable Diseases," *Med. Hist.* 21:61-68, 1977.

The classical paper on the position of contagion in the thinking of physicians in the first half of the nineteenth century is by E. H. Ackerknecht, "Anticontagionism Between 1821 and 1867," *Bull. Hist. Med.* 22:562-593, 1948. A number of Ackerknecht's more important positions, at least as they apply to England, have been challenged by M. Pelling in *Cholera, Fever and English Medicine, 1825-1865*, London: Oxford University Press, 1978.

The story of Semmelweis generally follows W. J. Sinclair, *Semmelweis: His Life and His Doctrine*, Manchester: University of Manchester Press, 1909. The academic and political strife occasioned by Semmelweis's actions have been chronicled by E. Lesky, *Ignaz Phillip Semmelweis und die Wiener Medezinische Schule*, Wein: Kommissionsverlag der Osterreichischen Akademie der Wissenschaften, 1964. Semmelweis's principal work, *Kindbettkiebers*, has been translated into English by F. P. Murphy, *Medical Classics*, Baltimore: Williams and Wilkins Company, vol. 5, 1941.

The animalcular theory is elucidated by Bulloch (see above); by C.E.A. Winslow in *The Conquest of Epidemic Disease*, Princeton, N.J.: Princeton University Press, 1943; and, in its earlier history, by C. Singer and D. Singer, "The Development of the Doctrine of Contagium Vivum, 1500-1750," *History of Medicine Section* (Seventeenth International Congress of Medicine, 1913), London: Oxford University Press, 1914.

Pasteur biographies include R. Vallery-Radot, *The Life of Pasteur*, New York: Doubleday, Page & Company, 1916, and R. Dubos, *Louis Pasteur: Free Lance of Science*, Boston: Little, Brown & Company, 1950. The reader desiring a more current estimate should consult the excellent piece by G. Geison in the *Dictionary of Scientific Biography*, New York: Charles Scribner's Sons, 1974, vol. 10, pp. 350-416. Lister's story is told by, among many others, D. Guthrie in *Lord Lister: His Life and Doctrine*, Baltimore: Williams and Wilkins Company, 1949.

The spontaneous generation debate has been greatly clarified in recent years by J. Farley and G. L. Geison, "Science, Politics and Spontaneous Generation in Nineteenth Century France: The Pasteur-Pouchet Debate," *Bull. Hist. Med.* 46:161-198, 1974, and by J. Farley, *The Spontaneous Generation Controversy from Descartes to Oparin*, Baltimore: Johns Hopkins University Press, 1974.

There is no definitive biography of Koch in English. For a translation of many of his own thoughts on matters relevant to this chapter, see Lechevalier and Solotorovsky. Bulloch nicely describes the problems involved in cultivating bacteria. Koch's obligations to his mentor, Henle, are found in G. Rosen, "Jacob

Henle: On Miasmata and Contagia," *Bull. Inst. Hist. Med.* 6:907-983, 1938. The evolution of the original postulates has been traced by A. S. Evans, "Causation and Disease: The Henle-Koch Postulates Revisited," *Yale J. Biol. and Med.* 49:175-195, 1976.

Good summaries on the germ theory's acceptance and influence in the United States are provided by P. A. Richmond, "American Attitudes Toward the Germ Theory of Disease, 1860-1880," *J. Hist. Med.* 9:428-454, 1954, and G. H. Brieger, "American Surgery and the Germ Theory of Disease," *Bull. Hist. Med.* 40:135-145, 1966.

9
SPECIFIC
PREVENTION

To this point we have developed the main lines leading to our current understanding of the nature and cause of disease and its diagnosis. One of the more important generalizations in this regard is that our conception of disease tends to determine our attempts to deal with it. If you believe congenital syphilis spreads from mother to child by a microscopic organism capable of crossing the placental barrier and highly sensitive to a chemical called penicillin, you are not likely to treat the condition with exhortations to the gods. As a rule then, in medicine concepts dictate actions, and the actions in this case are those directed at controlling disease through prevention and therapy.

Prevention has always been the ideal of medicine, and paradoxically the least attended to in practice. Most of the accomplishments in the prevention of disease have come through administrative and legislative channels, through public health departments, and from laws such as those demanding immunization of school children. Neither physicians nor patients in the Western world have paid much more than lip service to these efforts. Physicians, for their part, have been disease and treatment oriented because of a longstanding emphasis in their educational process and because treating a case of typhoid fever is more challenging than properly placing a privy. Patients, for their part, are not always willing to make the changes in living patterns which would help prevent the chronic degenerative and malignant diseases that have become the source of our main morbidity and mortality.

To extend Claude Bernard's physiological conception, it might be said that disease is preventable by altering either the external or internal environment. Swamps can be drained to eliminate the yellow fever mosquito, or a vaccine can be injected to enhance the body's immune response should it encounter the virus of yellow fever. The division into external (or environmental, as it will be called here) and internal prevention is historically appropriate because the two approaches developed along distinctly separate lines and did not merge effectively until the arrival of the present century.

Environmental Prevention from Antiquity to the Mid-Eighteenth Century

Public health among the ancient Hebrews has been mentioned. That of Greece and Rome will occupy us only in passing, since we know so little about it. We know that the public medical function was overseen by magistrates and rulers, who hired physicians for public service, but we know almost nothing of the daily activities of these early workers. The Romans are remembered for the excellence of their water supply, sewage disposal system, and baths, but much of this was based on esthetic and other cultural influences and involved no conscious attempt to prevent disease. On empirical grounds, however, it appears that the Romans did make a connection between swampy marshes and certain diseases, notably malaria, and accordingly emphasized the importance of careful selection of building sites for farms and cities.

Steps taken in public health during the Middle Ages belie the notion that this was a period of pervasive intellectual and social torpidity. Particularly from the twelfth century on, the idea developed that society collectively had a special responsibility for the lame and the halt, a belief that was translated into the widespread development of hospitals. Public health boards in the modern sense did not exist, but the council system that had developed for the administration of community affairs in general, also involved itself in the protection of the common health.

The bubonic plague of the fourteenth century convinced almost everyone of the contagiousness of disease and in turn focussed attention on attempts at prevention. One aspect of this was a general attack on filth. Streets were cleaned and regulations enacted against emptying cesspools and keeping pigs. In England in 1388 the first laws against general nuisances were passed. The plague also gave impetus to the practice of quarantine. As early as A.D. 1000 Venice was employing administrators to control maritime sanitation, but only on an ad hoc basis as each new epidemic broke out. The period of detention was extended to thirty days and later to forty, the latter giving us the origin of the word quarantine. But there was no quarantining the rats, as we have seen; plague returned time and again into the eighteenth century.

The burgeoning of science, a hallmark of the Renaissance centuries, conferred little practical benefit on those interested in the prevention of disease. An exception here was the city-states of Northern Italy. Beginning with the first major outbreak of bubonic plague during 1347–1348, which convinced physicians and laymen alike that the disease was highly contagious, Venice established a health board, which became permanent after 1527. The innovation spread to other cities, and Italy was soon far ahead of the rest of Europe in matters of public health. By the middle of the sixteenth century the boards, which were generally under nonphysician control, had spread their jurisdictions beyond control of epidemic disease to include foodstuffs; water supplies; sewers; cemeteries; the routines of physicians, surgeons, and apothecaries; and the activities of beggars and prostitutes. All in all it was a remarkable chapter in the history of preventive medicine, and one that has been generally overlooked.

The basic question remains: Did this early example of excellent public health organization have any real effect on morbidity and mortality from contagious diseases? In an ultimate sense no answer is possible. For that, we would have to rerun the same segment of history without the presence of the health boards. In all likelihood the final impact of the combined measures of prevention was small. This is because the principals lacked information about the crucial role of rats in spreading plague. In the outbreak of 1656–1657, for example, Genoa lost 5,500 of its 73,000 citizens, a toll which led the superintendent of the principal pesthouse to wonder, if no preventive measures had been taken, would Genoa have suffered even more severely?

Still, this early chapter in Northern Italy demonstrated the role that effective administration would have to assume in the centuries that followed. It also revealed the conflicts that would become important again during the Sanitary Movement of the nineteenth century, disputes that seem always to arise when public health measures are perceived as inimical to economic interests or individual liberties.

In the seventeenth century two developments deserve mention. The first, the influence of the English physician Thomas Sydenham, has already been touched on. Sydenham, in extolling the notion of the epidemic constitution, called proper attention to the role of the seasons in human disease. But whatever contribution to epidemiology he made thereby was more than offset by the negative influence he had on thinking about contagion generally. Reportedly he mentions contagion definitely in only three places in his writing, and these with regard to plague and venereal disease. Thus he did not discuss the communicability of disease even where measles and smallpox were concerned. His influence on his contemporaries apparently was not as great as it became in later decades, when it must have directed many away from thinking in terms of contagion.

The seventeenth century saw the expansion of mercantilism, and with it an interest in numbers that had not existed before. The ultimate goal of mercantilism was more power for the state. At bottom this meant a favorable balance of trade in a rapidly expanding colonial world. At home a major emphasis was placed on increasing the population under a government which in turn was responsible for the material well-being of all. Ultimately health came to be viewed as an important aspect of governmental responsibility. But this would come about only when it was demonstrated that the governing systems were failing in this particular duty, and for that, accurate vital statistics were needed.

The importance of what has been called "political arithmetic" was recognized by authorities as early as the Italian Renaissance, but the individual who coined the term and placed health in the political calculus was the English physician and political economist Sir William Petty (1623-1687). Repeatedly Petty emphasized the crucial importance of a healthy citizenry in the furtherance of the power of the state. His lead was exploited by his friend John Graunt (1620-1674), who published the first ambitious study of mortality figures in his 1662 *Natural and Political Observations Made upon the Bills of Mortality.* From his study of deaths in London during the twenty years before 1658, Graunt drew four main conclusions. He demonstrated that certain diseases, such as consumptions, dropsies, gout, and suicide, had a nearly constant mortality; that is, they produced almost identical percentages of death year after year. He demonstrated that more males were born each year than females, although a higher death rate in males evened out the ratio as years passed. He found that rural death rates were lower than those of city dwellers, and finally, he called attention to the inordinately high mortality among infants and children.

On the lighter side Graunt also concluded that "the irreligious proposals of some, to multiply people by Polygamy" was not a reasonable solution to the state's need for a larger population, that the notion that the entry of kings caused epidemics of plague was "false and seditious," that London was "perhaps a Head too big for the Body" of England, and that the streets as they were could not accommodate the daily traffic of coaches.[1]

In concluding his small book Graunt asked, "To what purpose tends all this labourious bustling and groping?" He went on to show that there is more to such work than the juggling of figures. Simply put, he argued that the state cannot govern properly in the absence of accurate information – statistics – on all aspects of the realm, but particularly on its citizens.

Graunt was neither scientist nor physician, but a draper by trade. He had been elected to the Royal Society after his book appeared in 1662, but when the society was reorganized under the charter of Charles II of 1663, the propriety of including a lowly draper in the company of Olympians was questioned. The matter was not long debated; King Charles promptly advised the society "that if they found any more such tradesmen they should be sure to admit them without more ado."[2]

Petty and Graunt had made a good start, the one by advocating

the theoretical importance of political arithmetic, the other by
drawing significant conclusions from the existing Bills of Mortality, however faulty and incomplete. Their work could not be
translated directly into improved public health largely because
in the seventeenth century public and governmental interest was
not yet sufficient to bring about the necessary administrative
structure. Indeed, for most of the eighteenth century public
health matters would rest in the hands of local councils which
were direct descendants of those arising in the later Middle
Ages. During this period, however, the commonwealth advocated by Thomas Hobbes in his *Leviathan* was gradually emerging; localized rule was gradually yielding to the larger modern
state.

The responsibility for health matters incumbent on the new
state – this merger of mercantilism and absolute monarchy as it
occurred in Germany – would be spelled out at the end of the
eighteenth century by the physician Johann Peter Frank
(1745–1821). Frank, who personifies the paternalistic approach
to public health, was influenced in his sweeping outlook by a
first-hand exposure to the organization and tradition of public
health in Northern Italy mentioned earlier. To his mind citizens,
however well intentioned, were ultimately children. They must
be told what was best for their health, and it devolved on the
state to see that right was done. Frank put forth his ideas in meticulous detail in six volumes between 1779 and 1817 in a labor
entitled *System einer völlstandigen medizinischen Polizei* (A System
of Complete Medical Police). The title accurately reflects the contents. It was the first detailed health program of the sort that
would now be labeled "womb to tomb." Prenatal and perinatal
care, infant and child health, hygiene in the schools, food, clothing, recreation, housing, rescue, sewage and garbage disposal,
water supply, maintenance of public comfort stations – all were
there as one comprehensive health policy to be orchestrated,
right down to the finest tuning, by benevolent governmental
bureaucrats.

The lengths to which Frank was willing to go in controlling the
citizen's activities for his own welfare would offend today's civil
libertarians as readily as they did John Stewart Mill. In one
amusing section Frank urged authorities to limit the duration of

balls and to proscribe certain erotic dances such as the waltz. Parents were admonished to protect their daughters against such rampant pleasures, particularly during their menstrual periods, and to enforce a half-hour's rest after the end of dancing before letting the young people depart.

Though many of Frank's prescriptions strike us as unacceptable now, his present importance lies in the value he placed on a healthy citizenry, a repeatedly expressed goal of the sanitary reformers of the nineteenth century.

The Nineteenth Century: Sanitary Reform

Frank's last book in his six-volume series appeared in the nineteenth century. During the first forty years of that century neither the philosophy of the Enlightenment nor the enlightened absolutism advocated by Frank had much practical effect on the health of the masses. But both approaches, and the discussions they generated, helped set the stage for the movement that dominated the middle decades of the nineteenth century, the salutary saga of sanitary reform.

The living habits of Western Europeans and Americans before the period of decent sanitation are almost too grim to convey to a modern reader by the written word. Since, to the sanitary reformers, filth itself and not some tiny animals caused disease, it is important to understand the abysmal scenes they encountered when they finally took a firsthand look at the surroundings of the working class and unemployed.

The satirist Jonathan Swift has given us a few lines to illustrate conditions during that period known as the Enlightenment.

> Now from all parts the swelling kennels flow,
> And bear their trophies with them as they go;
> Filth of all hues and odors seem to tell
> What street they sailed from by the sight and smell;
> Sweepings from the butchers' stalls, dung, guts and blood,
> Drowned puppies, stinking sprats, all drenched in muck,
> Dead cats and turnip-top come tumbling down the flood.[3]

Conditions within the home were little better than those of the street. The same clothing might be worn for months or even years, a practice that had gone on for centuries. With no internal plumbing or efficient way of heating water, bathing understandably was considered an ordeal. Even after stoves were invented, we find one young man inquiring with revealing anxiety, "I have been in the habit during the past winter of taking a warm bath every three weeks. Is this too often to follow year round?"[4]

As the nineteenth century progressed, the steam engine and its product, the Industrial Revolution, along with a general rise in population after 1750, brought hordes of rural inhabitants to the cities. To accommodate this rising tide, substandard housing was rapidly erected and existing homes became increasingly crowded. Of some 2,500 cellars surveyed in Manchester in the mid-nineteenth century, one bed accommodated three persons in 1,500 instances; 738 slept four; and 281, five. Things were no better in the United States. In New York's Cherry Street, for example, a five-story tenement held 120 families, totaling more than 500 persons.

The effects of such conditions, compounded many times as the Industrial Revolution spread and grew, were bound to be reflected in the stark figures of the bills of mortality. The death rate in New York City was 21 per 1,000 in 1810 and 37 per 1,000 in 1857, an increase of more than 75 percent in slightly less than half a century. The same general picture prevailed in Britain and to a lesser extent in Germany, where industrialization was late arriving.

The final piece to be placed on the stage of the sanitary reformers was the changing popular and official view of cleanliness itself. Up to and throughout the eighteenth century, cleanliness was not associated primarily with health. Bathing originated largely for esthetic purposes and only gradually took on the aspect of a moral and religious obligation. It was not until the end of the eighteenth century that what has been termed a physiological concept of cleanliness began gaining ground, once again to be reinforced by moral overtones. Thus in the developing nineteenth century a certain irony emerged—at the same time the working classes were beginning to associate cleanliness with health, they were being forced by social conditions into the structured filth of the slums.

Cholera, the Catalyst

The need for improved public health became obvious to many as the excesses of the Industrial Revolution agglomerated through the first decades of the nineteenth century in Britain. But the working class, as was usual at the time, was powerless to effect any large environmental reform. For change to occur, the poor required aid from the upper and ruling classes. The latter, seldom dilatory in perceiving their own best interests, suddenly became more sensitive to the needs of the poor as the diseases of the hovels threatened to spread to the manors. The principal catalyst in this regard was cholera.

Cholera is an acute infectious disease caused by a comma-shaped bacterium, the *Vibrio cholerae*. The best evidence at this time indicates that the disease first appeared in the West in 1830. Victims acquire cholera by ingesting food or drink contaminated by the feces of those suffering the disease or acting as carriers. The chief symptom and cause of death is a profuse diarrhea of up to seven quarts or more in the first twenty-four hours. The diarrhea is due to a toxin produced by the bacterium, and the fluid lost contains large quantities of sodium, potassium, and bicarbonate, depletions which, if unchecked, lead to death. The cholera bacillus is readily killed by tetracycline antibiotics, and if the lost salts and water are replaced the mortality is near zero.

None of this, of course, was known during the three great visitations of cholera in the nineteenth century, when in contrast to scurvy as the scourge of the seafaring man, cholera became known as the scourge of nations. From its ageless home in India, major epidemics of cholera struck England in 1831, 1848, and 1865, on each occasion reaching the United States one year later. The mortality rate among those contracting the disease ran to about 50 percent, but because persons with normal gastric acidity are largely protected against the disease, the overall incidence was often lower than 1 percent of the population. Despite its low incidence cholera remained particularly fearsome because of its explosive nature. In the epidemic of the early 1830s some 7,000 Parisians died in eighteen days, while Glasgow had 228 deaths in a single week. Still, the overall mortality scarcely counted as a demographic threat. The total deaths for the four major outbreaks in England and Wales were some 21,000 in 1831–1832; 53,000 in 1849, 20,000 in 1854, and 14,000 in 1866.

The importance of cholera for the purpose at hand is the impetus it gave public health endeavors in the United States and Britain. The association between cholera mortality and poor living conditions was soon too obvious to be ignored. At the same time, the disease demonstrated that it could reach the affluent as well. This led to the accelerated interest among governmental officials and the wealthy in the plight of the working man and unemployed that has been seen as the beginnings of the modern public health movement. In making this conclusion, however, it should be kept in mind that the influence of cholera on public health policy was neither immediate nor direct. On the contrary, as the 1832 epidemic waned in Britain, a distinct complacency set in. The mortality had not been as great as feared; the well-to-do had not been heavily attacked; and the medical profession had not been able to derive any significant lessons of causation or prevention. The result was that little sanitary reform ensued, and indeed, the Public Health Acts of 1848 probably related more to fear of typhus than cholera. The influence of the 1832 outbreak was instead indirect and remote. It included increased knowledge and confidence on the part of physicians who would encounter the disease later in the century, but above all, it was carried in the personal experiences of young men who would, upon attaining position and influence, take the lead in the sanitary reform that finally occurred.

Sanitary Reform, 1840–1880

In terms of personalities, the origins of sanitary reform in Britain can be carried back to Jeremy Bentham (1748–1832), even though he played no direct part. Bentham brought to the nineteenth century the aspirations of the French Encyclopedists, which had been thwarted by the Revolution of 1789. He was convinced that a proper blend of governmental intervention and restraint could lead human beings to do what was best for themselves, individually and collectively. One of Bentham's disciples, Edwin Chadwick (1800–1890), extended this line of reasoning to the then novel idea that man had the wherewithal to shape his environment, more specifically to eliminate the diseases of filth by doing away with the filth. Before this process could begin, of course, it was necessary to demonstrate a causal relationship between living conditions and disease. To this end Chadwick and his colleagues labored for three years before bringing out in 1842 their monumental *Sanitary Condition of the Labouring Population of Great Britain.* In this Chadwick demonstrated repeatedly and convincingly that disease was related to income, habitat, and working conditions. The book contained the essence of what would come to be called the Great Sanitary Awakening.

Chadwick was not a medical man, but as his movement gained momentum, a number of physicians became involved in the effort. One of these, John Simon (1816-1904), took over leadership of the sanitary program from Chadwick. For some twenty years he functioned as one of the most effective health educators of all time. In the United States physicians played leadership roles from the outset, and at times medical societies functioned as boards of health. The enactment of the New York Metropolitan Health Bill of 1866 was a crucial victory for that city and has been viewed as a turning point for the United States at large.

The Great Sanitary Awakening can be placed in the forty years between 1840 and 1880 — although, in a sense, it has never ended. It was a remarkable, but by no means unique, example of doing the right thing for the wrong reason. The filth theory of disease, after all, had no basis in scientific fact. It was little more than a revival of the ancient doctrine of miasm, although admittedly now buttressed with statistical and epidemiological evidence. But the important fact remains that the actions that followed subscription to the theory did help control disease. The evidence for this is largely inferential; that is, the incidence of a number of contagious diseases began declining before anything was known of their cause, treatment, or prevention.

The positive results of the sanitary movement could not be explained until after the discoveries of bacteriology in the last two decades of the nineteenth century. The episode proves once more that at times disease can be controlled without understanding much of its nature. John Snow (1813-1858) effected a decrease in mortality during the 1854 cholera epidemic in London without knowing exactly what he was doing. In an elegant epidemiological study, he demonstrated that certain water supplies were producing many cases of cholera and others only a few. His efforts led to the removal of one such public pump handle on Broad Street, and the epidemic, already declining, soon abated altogether. It must be acknowledged parenthetically that Snow's achievement had little immediate effect on medical thinking, but his figures convinced William Farr (1807–1883) at the Registrar-General's office, and prepared him for the work that substantiated Snow's suspicions when cholera returned in 1865. Snow, however, was so much under the influence of the filth doctrine that when he first examined the water from the Broad Street pump and found it clear he was reluctant to condemn it. It remained for bacteriological knowledge to demonstrate finally that pure water meant nothing more than water free of germs and toxins, and that everything else was a matter of esthetics.

It has been said that the official reports issued by John Simon in the third quarter of the nineteenth century reflect almost perfectly the development of epidemiological theory between 1849 and 1878. At the outset of sanitary reform, disease was approached under an unrefined form of the old miasmatic doctrine. Due to the work of Snow and William Budd (1811–1880), who in 1856 did for typhoid fever what Snow had done for cholera seven years earlier, the importance of water in the spread of disease was gradually appreciated. As the dawn of bacteriology approached, it began to be appreciated that filth was the agent of disease and not the source itself. And finally, with Koch and Pasteur and their followers, the cause of contagious diseases was pinned to living, multiplying microorganisms. At that point, efforts at controlling the external environment finally began to be placed on a rational basis. It must be said in passing that the merging of understanding between the filth fighters and bacteriologists was not easy and automatic. A number of sanitarians remained openly hostile to the methods and findings of the "New Science" in the last half of the nineteenth century. In any ultimate sense it is difficult to assess the overall effects of the sanitary movement. Cholera did not return to Western Europe after 1866, and certainly one would expect liquid-borne diseases such as typhoid and the typhus transmitted by the body louse to decrease in incidence with general improvements in hygiene. The problem, as we shall see in a later chapter, is one of assigning causality. A number of other factors, such as improved nutrition, were no doubt at play in ways that cannot be sorted out with any feeling of confidence.

Specific Prevention and the Internal Environment

The most rigorous imaginable environmental control will never do away with all human contagions. A number of infectious diseases spread directly from human to human and have no vulnerable points in their life cycle that can be attacked through an environmental approach. Examples of such diseases are measles, mumps, infectious mononucleosis, and poliomyelitis. Prevention here depends on altering the immune system so that when the inevitable meeting occurs between microbe and man, few or no symptoms result. Further, certain groups of organisms are so widespread in our surroundings that elimination is practically out of the question. These include staphylococci, streptococci, and meningococci. For some of these there is no immunization, and control presently depends upon treatment after symptoms have appeared.

For the Western world since the seventeenth century, smallpox has been among the most important contagious diseases not amenable to manipulation of the external environment. Smallpox is a highly contagious viral disease transmitted by respiratory droplets or direct contact with crusts on the infected blisters (pustules). The disease is feared on two scores, the mortality itself and the severe scarring (pocking), caused by deep intradermal penetration of the pustules. A full-blown attack generally confers lifelong immunity.

The mortality associated with smallpox was terrible enough even bearing in mind the deficiencies of mortality bills in the earlier periods. If contemporary reports can be believed for seventeenth-century England, one of four died of the disease and half the population was disfigured by pockmarks. The same dismal reports persisted until the end of the eighteenth century, when the average annual deaths from the disease were put at

40,000 for the United Kingdom and 3,000 for London alone. Even as late as 1871–1872, a century or so after the disease was theoretically controllable, an epidemic of smallpox carried off 42,000 persons in England and Wales. Of the reign of terror accompanying these recurrent incursions, Macaulay wrote, in describing the death of Mary in his *History of England:*

The smallpox was always present, filling the church-yards with corpses, tormenting with constant fears all whom it had not yet stricken, leaving on those whose lives it spared the hideous traces of its power, turning the babe into a changeling at which the mother shuddered, and making the eyes and cheeks of the betrothed maiden objects of horror to the lover.[5]

Unlike the diseases of filth, smallpox was no respecter of persons. Queen Anne was badly pocked; Charles I lost two children; and Queen Mary II died of the disease. For this reason it was bound to be written of more than, say, typhoid or typhus. The democratic quality of smallpox led to a resignation in the face of death and loss that is missing from the current scene, in which all concerned act as though death is alien to the cycle of life. The earlier stoical acceptance of death from disease, even premature death, led to the many almost casual accounts of loss of children that the modern reader finds at once poignant and puzzling. Montaigne in later life was quoted as saying, "I lost two or three children as nurslings, not without regret but without great grief."[6]

Phase One: Variolation

Unknown to Westerners in the eighteenth century, smallpox had long been a preventable disease. For centuries a practice that would come to be called ingrafting or inoculation or variolation had been practiced in Russia, India, China, and Africa. Variolation consisted of introducing into a susceptible person a small amount of pus from an active case of smallpox. In different times and places it was done by rubbing the material into the mucous membranes of the nose, or introducing it directly into the blood stream through an opened vein. Later, in a quest for added safety, a method was developed in which the skin was punctured, but without direct placement of the pus in the bloodstream. Whatever the method, the goal was to produce a minor attack of the disease and thus permanent immunity.

Rumors of smallpox inoculation reached England between 1675 and 1714. During the next seven years several investigations and communications to the Royal Society convinced English physicians that inoculation actually was being performed in other lands but left them skeptical of the efficacy of the undertaking, at least for Englishmen. Due in part to the audacity of Lady Mary Montagu (1689–1762) and the efforts of physicians such as Hans Sloane (1660–1753), a few inoculations took place, but reaction set in following two deaths that were apparently related to the variolation. At that point news reached London of a statistically successful inoculation experiment in Boston, and from that time on, confidence in the safety and effectiveness of variolation gradually rose in Europe as well as colonial America, North and South.

Phase Two: Vaccination

In capable hands smallpox inoculation was a relatively safe operation. Still, there was no escaping the fact that live smallpox virus was being transferred from the sick to the healthy, and the amount and virulency of the virus could not be controlled with anything resembling scientific precision. Individual deaths occurred, and it is even likely that epidemics resulted. The latter is difficult to establish, because inoculation campaigns usually awaited an announcement that an epidemic was imminent. Lady Mary Montagu's refusal to inoculate her daughter because her nurse had never had smallpox reflects the general recognition that the operation carried a measure of danger. By the time inoculation was firmly established in Britain, a new and safer method was announced there by a medical practitioner of Berkeley, Edward Jenner (1749–1823).

In Jenner's region a popular notion existed that those who had suffered a bout of cowpox were forever immune to the smallpox, an immensely important phenomenon if it was true, because cowpox was a relatively mild disease, rarely fatal even in severe instances. If it somehow provided a natural cross-immunity to smallpox, it followed that artificially induced cowpox would avoid the dangers of inoculation. Apparently Jenner had mentioned all this while under the tutelage of the great John Hunter, the man who demonstrated the potential of experimentation in surgery. Hunter was not much intrigued at the time, but his later advice to Jenner would prove sound. "Do not think," he reportedly said, "but try; be patient, be accurate."[7]

In his first experimental step Jenner found that those who had been through the cowpox did not suffer even the usual mild case when inoculated for smallpox. As he gained experience of this sort, he decided to follow Hunter's advice and take a more direct approach. On May 14, 1796, he took material from a cowpox lesion from a dairymaid and inserted it into the arm of a young boy by means of two half-inch incisions that barely penetrated the superficial layer of the skin. On the following July 1, Jenner challenged the boy with a dose of smallpox pus, encountering no untoward effects.

With this and similar data he wrote for permission to present his findings to the Royal Society, but was admonished that he should think twice before claiming anything so alien to existing knowledge, and so incredible in any event. In adopting this stance it should be emphasized that the society was not enshrouding itself in mindless conservatism. Jenner's conclusions were indeed incredible. No instance was recognized in which a largely animal disease could protect human beings from a different disease, and the most fearsome of the time at that. Further, the number of cases he presented was small, nor was there any way to be certain that his successful cases had not gained previous immunity from mild cases of smallpox or even a forgotten inoculation in childhood. But Jenner's character featured a persistence bordering on stubbornness. He was convinced of the essential accuracy of his observations, and so in 1798 he published his findings and conclusions under his own sponsorship. The book, known familiarly as the *Inquiry*, carried the burdensome title of *An Inquiry into the Causes and Effects of the Variolae Vaccinae, A Disease Discovered in Some of the Western Counties of England, Particularly Gloucestershire, and Known by the Name of the Cowpox*. Jenner's method was termed vaccination by a surgeon in Plymouth, and later, as a gesture of appreciation to Jenner, Louis Pasteur would adopt the word to describe the general process of artificially inducing immunization.

By 1786, almost a half-century after the advent of inoculation in the West, London stations set up to serve the public reportedly had inoculated only 6,581 persons. In contrast to the slow progress of variolation, Jenner's vaccination spread rapidly, and the results were not long in appearing. Even after the spread of inoculation, the estimate is that London suffered an average of 3,000 smallpox deaths annually in the fifty years before Jenner's announcement. In 1800, two years after Jenner published, the figure was 2,409. By 1802 deaths had dropped to 1,173 and by 1804 to 622.

Impressive as these figures appear in retrospect, by no means did they hand Jenner an uncontested victory. As the nineteenth century progressed, opposition to vaccination remained, and it was particularly heated in countries where compulsion was sought through legal means. But it was to be enforced vaccination, such as that adopted in Britain in 1853, that finally eradicated doubts about the efficacy of vaccination, even though the issue of civil liberties remained. In 1870 a smallpox pandemic swept the globe, lasting from three to five years. Four countries having compulsory vaccination at the time had an average of 338 deaths per one million persons during the five years after 1870. The figure in four equally industrialized countries without compulsory vaccination was 1,141, or more than three times as high. Such differences, repeated time and again, gradually shifted the balance against the antivaccinationists. The final chapter in this story brings us into strictly modern times. In 1980, after more than two years during which no new natural cases were reported, the World Health Organization declared smallpox, as Jenner had ventured to hope, "extirpated from the earth."

Pasteur and Specific Prevention

In the ordinary course of scientific development, a discovery which was perceived as momentous in its time, as Jenner's was, might be expected to set off a flurry of investigation leading to artificial immunizations against other diseases. In truth Jenner's lead turned out to be a cul-de-sac. His discovery depended on a natural fluke of sorts, on the fact that a virus that caused a relatively innocuous human disease, cowpox, provided cross-immunity to the deadly smallpox. It would be a benign Nature indeed that furnished similar circumstances for all the important contagious diseases confronting mankind. To put it another way, the older inoculation model held more promise than did that of the vaccination that replaced it. Inoculation utilized an attenuated form of the same microbe that caused the disease in question, coupled with an unnatural method of producing a mild infection, that is, injection into the skin or bloodstream. Variolation, then, at least in theory, held the promise of universality, while vaccination was limited to a single disease.

Historically the matter developed exactly along these lines; no new examples of cross-immunity surfaced in the years after Jenner. On the other hand, attempts to immunize by inoculation had taken place long before vaccination was popularized. In 1759 an Edinburgh physician, Francis Home (1719–1813), reported his attempts at controlling measles "in the same way that the Turks had taught us to mitigate the Small Pox." Since the measles eruption is not fluid-filled as is smallpox, Home used the blood of infected individuals to transfer the protection. He managed to secure thirteen volunteers for these mini-transfusions, and although he was satisfied that he had succeeded, the method failed to attract a medical or popular following. In all probability he was not accomplishing what he hoped, and certainly there was danger from infection and allergic reactions in such a crude approach.

But Home's venture was nothing compared to the disaster inherent in the mid-nineteenth-century proposal considered by the Paris Academy of Medicine. Here the plan was to vaccinate the whole of French youth against syphilis. A principal proponent of this plan was one Joseph-Alexandre Auzias-Turenne (1812–1870), who drew his inspiration from Jenner's success with smallpox vaccination. In Auzias-Turenne's mistaken thinking, the lesion called a soft chancre was an attenuated form of the hard chancre, the primary lesion of syphilis. By injecting material from a soft chancre, he reasoned, the recipient would be protected against syphilis just as recipients of cowpox were protected against smallpox. We now know that soft chancre is an early manifestation of an entirely different disease, chancroid, and has little in common with syphilis beyond the venereal mode of spread. Chancroid is caused by a bacterium *Hemophilus ducreyi*, and syphilis by the spirochete *Treponema pallidum*, between which there is no cross-immunity whatever. Had Auzias-Turenne prevailed on the powers of France to proceed with his plan, untold thousands of French youths presumably would have been given chancroid simultaneously with an imaginary immunity to syphilis. Still, his failure did not consign Auzias-Turenne to total oblivion. His ideas published in *La Syphilisation* in 1878 came to the attention of, and perhaps reinforced, the thinking of the man who was to place immunization on a scientific basis, Louis Pasteur.

When we left Pasteur, it may be recalled, he had not turned his full attention to human disease. In part this was because he was, as he put it, a stranger to medical and veterinary knowledge. As we return our attention to his activities, however, he is involved in work that will shift his full attention to the prevention of disease in animals and man.

In the spring of 1879 Pasteur was working with cholera in chickens. The lapse in work occasioned by a summer vacation produced for Pasteur another example of the phenomenon of serendipity. Returning to his experiments, Pasteur found that the samples of chicken cholera microbes that had languished in their incubators over the summer would not induce cholera as they had before. When he grew a new culture of cholera bacilli and injected it into these same chickens, as well as some he had freshly procured, Pasteur met an unexpected result. The new chickens died of cholera as expected; those which had been injected first with the old, then with the new cholera growths, survived. In some way the virulence of the old cultures had diminished over the summer. Perhaps drawing on his knowledge of Jenner's work, which had long intrigued him, Pasteur perceived the relationship between his attenuated cholera bacilli and Jenner's cowpox. He also recognized a crucial difference of the highest importance. In theory at least, his model was applicable to any microorganism which could be isolated and cultured. Virulence might be reduced by heating, cooling, chemicals, successive passages through the appropriate animals, by any number of means. If the results followed those of the chicken cholera, he would have a microorganism which could not produce serious disease, but which could still trigger the immune system in a way that would protect the animal against the next encounter with a fully virulent germ of the same type.

Pasteur was quick to demonstrate the truth and practical implications of his new discovery. On February 28, 1881, he announced the development of a vaccine for anthrax, and at the same time he laid out his basic tenet that bacterial virulence was not a fixed attribute but could be developed at many points on a given scale. Later that year, in the face of many doubters, he staged his famous large-scale experiment at Pouilly le Fort, in which thirty-one farm animals protected with his vaccine survived an injection of anthrax, while all the control sheep and the single goat died and the four control cows became ill. "In the multitude at Pouilly le Fort, that day," it was said, "there were no longer any skeptics but only admirers."[8] Gradually the same would be said of the scientific community at large. Within four years Pasteur had demonstrated the versatility of his model by creating vaccines against chicken cholera, anthrax, swine erysipelas, and rabies.

Specific Prevention in the Twentieth Century

In the first half of the nineteenth century, the sanitarians had silenced the contagionists with one reason above all. Vague though it was, the concept of disease from filth was more concrete than the evidence available to those championing infection. In the last part of the century the tables were turned, and the public health movement was eclipsed by the dramatic discoveries of the new bacteriology now coming "like corn popping in a pan."[9] On balance, however, the bacteriological revelations did nothing more than demonstrate that the sanitarians had been right for the wrong reasons. The advent of vaccines and antitoxins did not detract from the need for public hygiene. On the contrary, efforts to control the external environment were now finally based in rationality. At last it was clear why the outhouse had to be physically distant from the well, and why tuberculars should not spit on the sidewalk.

In the twentieth century, efforts at controlling the external and internal environment gradually merged under the general aegis of preventive medicine. At the same time the concept of specific prevention was broadened into areas other than those devoted to contagious diseases, and the movement became international in scope. One result was a massive program of public education in schools, churches, and elsewhere. From this came an unprecedented participation of people, even remotely located, in the wedding of the sanitary movement and the discoveries of bacteriology. In rural Fredonia, Kansas, on October 5, 1915, a "sanitary parade" took place. The governor and all the senators and congressmen of the state led the march.

Schools are closed; enthusiastic crowds have pushed into the town from miles around; trains leaving the city are held up so that visitors will not miss the parade. There are twenty-six floats, including a procession of undertakers in deep mourning at the coming of sanitation. A huge fly is dragging in its wake thirteen empty baby buggies, boys dressed in black robes have ropes around their necks held by Typhoid, the Lord High Executioner; all the hearses of Wilson County are participating, with each hearse containing an effigy of some disease caused by insanitary conditions. Was public health education ever made more forceful or meaningful? Would anyone presume to weigh the impact of these events on the impressionable minds of children?[10]

It is not easy to sort out with any hope of precision the relative roles played by the sanitary movement and the rise of bacteriology and immunology in the eradication of contagious diseases. One point, nevertheless, can be restated with certainty: many of the more important infectious diseases were already declining before the advent of either specific causation or artificial immunization. Among these were typhoid, typhus, tuberculosis, malaria, and yellow fever. Add to this smallpox, for which specific prevention was available, and it becomes clear that prevention, not treatment, has been the major factor in reducing human suffering and death from disease. The reduction has been remarkable given the short time involved. In 1900 only 13 million (18 percent) of the population of the United States was over forty-five years of age. A half-century later the figure was 43 million people, or 30 percent of the population. The chief reason for this increase was reduction in deaths from the contagious diseases of childhood. On the other hand, life expectancy itself has not been extended appreciably. The person reaching age forty-five can expect to live only about the same number of years as his counterpart of several decades ago.

An important feature of the figures just mentioned is a change in the pattern of diseases producing the bulk of mortality in industrialized societies. In 1900 the contagious diseases were far and away the most important. Today it is the chronic degenerative and malignant diseases, principally heart and respiratory disease, cancer, and stroke. Of these not enough is known either of causation or prevention. Deficient though it is, treatment stands as the main current approach, and it is the development of specific therapy that occupies us next.

Notes

1. Graunt, J. *Natural and Political Observations Made upon the Bills of Mortality.* London: John Martyn and James Allestry, 3rd ed., 1665, dedication.

2. Charles, J. *Research and Public Health.* London: Oxford University Press, 1961, p. 51.

3. Rosen, G. *A History of Public Health.* New York: MD Publications, 1958, p. 152.

4. Shryock, R. H. *Medicine in America: Historical Essays.* Baltimore: Johns Hopkins University Press, 1966, p. 114.

5. Clendening, L. *Source Book of Medical History.* New York: Paul B. Hoeber, Inc., 1942, p. 292.

6. Rosen, G. "Medicine as a Function of Society," in King, L. S. *Mainstreams of Medicine.* Austin: University of Texas Press, 1971, pp. 31-32.

7. Anon. *Brit. Med. J.* 2:5, July 5, 1902.

8. Dubos, R. J. *Louis Pasteur: Free Lance of Science.* Boston: Little, Brown & Company, 1950, p. 339.

9. Winslow, C.-E.A., quoting Harvey Cushing, *The Life of Hermann M. Biggs.* Philadelphia: Lea & Febiger, 1929, p. 60.

10. Bonner, T. N. *The Kansas Doctor.* Lawrence: University of Kansas Press, 1959, pp. 123-124.

Bibliographic Commentary

The single best overview of attempts to further health by controlling the external environment is G. Rosen, *A History of Public Health,* New York: MD Publications, 1958, which I have largely followed. Other valuable general works include C.-E.A. Winslow, *The Conquest of Epidemic Disease,* Princeton, N.J.: Princeton University Press, 1944; R. H. Shryock, *The Development of Modern Medicine,*

Madison: University of Wisconsin Press, 1979; and J. Charles, *Research and Public Health*, London: Oxford University Press, 1961. C. F. Brockington, *Public Health in the Nineteenth Century*, Edinburgh: E. & S. Livingston, 1965, includes many of the appropriate documents in full. For sketches of Chadwick and the other important persons in the public health movement, see M.E.M. Walker, *Pioneers of Public Health*, Freeport, N.Y.: Books for Libraries Press, 1930. There are now too many excellent accounts of local developments in public health to be listed here.

The story of the pioneering health boards of Northern Italy is recounted by C. M. Cipolla, *Public Health and the Medical Profession in the Renaissance*, Cambridge: Cambridge University Press, 1976.

The resistance of some sanitarians to the discoveries of bacteriologists and immunologists in the nineteenth century has been described in L. Stevenson, "Science down the Drain," *Bull. Hist. Med.* 29:1–26, 1955. American interest in "political arithmetic" is traced in J. H. Cassedy, *Demography in Early America: Beginnings of the Statistical Mind, 1600-1800*, Cambridge: Harvard University Press, 1969.

We finally have available in English extensive selections from J. P. Frank's principal work, along with an incisive introduction, in E. Lesky, *A System of Complete Medical Police*, Baltimore: Johns Hopkins University Press, 1976.

The development of cleanliness as a physiological concept follows O. Temkin, *The Double Face of Janus*, Baltimore: Johns Hopkins University Press, 1977, pp. 465–468.

There are now numerous solid accounts of the effects of cholera on society in general and the sanitary movement in particular. M. Pelling covers the English story in *Cholera, Fever and English Medicine 1825-1865*, Oxford: Oxford University Press, 1978. The American analysis is given by C. Rosenberg, *The Cholera Years: The United States in 1832, 1849, and 1866*, Chicago: University of Chicago Press, 1962, and by R. J. Morris, *Cholera 1832: The Social Response to an Epidemic*, New York: Holmes & Meier, 1976. A refreshing revision of persistent misconceptions in the history of cholera is that by N. Howard-Jones, "Choleranomalies: The Unhistory of Medicine as Exemplified by Cholera," *Perspectives Bio. and Med.* 15:422–433, 1972.

The story of inoculation is told by A. C. Klebs, "The Historic Evaluation of Variolation," *Bull. Johns Hopkins Hosp.* 24:69–83, 1913; R. P. Stearns, "Remarks upon the Introduction of Inoculation for Smallpox in England," *Bull. Hist. Med.* 24:103–122, 1950; J. B. Blake, "The Inoculation Controversy in Boston, 1721-1722," in J. W. Leavitt and R. L. Numbers, eds., *Sickness and Health in America: Readings in the History of Medicine and Public Health*, Madison: University of Wisconsin Press, 1978; O. T. Beall, Jr., and R. H. Shryock, *Cotton Mather: First Significant Figure in American Medicine*, Baltimore: Johns Hopkins Press, 1954; and above all, G. Miller, *The Adoption of Inoculation for Smallpox in England and France*, Philadelphia: University of Pennsylvania Press, 1957.

The role of Lady Montagu in the development of inoculation has been downgraded from its former place. In a story which has not been resolved to my satisfaction, the available evidence appears in R. Halsband, *The Life of Lady Mary Wortley Montagu*, Oxford: Clarendon Press, 1956; a later article by the same

author, "New Light on Lady Mary Wortley Montagu's Contribution to Inocula-
tion," *J. Hist. Med.* 8:390-405, 1953; and the latest word on the subject by G.
Miller, "Putting Lady Mary in Her Place: a Discussion of Historical Causation,"
Bull. Hist. Med. 55:2-16, 1981.

Jenner's classic is reproduced in C.N.B. Camac, *Classics of Medicine and Surgery,* New York: Dover Publications, 1959. His best biography is by D. Fisk, *Dr.
Jenner of Berkeley,* London: Heinemann, 1959. The combined effects of variolation and vaccination were studied in two articles, one by A. Newsholme and the
other by E. J. Edwardes, in *Brit. Med. J.* 2:17-30, 1902.

The fight against compulsory vaccination was far more vitriolic and effective
than today's compliant citizen might imagine. In this regard, see M. Kaufman,
"The American Anti-Vaccinationists and Their Arguments," *Bull. Hist. Med.*
41:463-478, 1967.

A controversy has developed in recent years over whether the vaccine materials employed by Jenner and the other early vaccinators were cowpox or an
attenuated form of smallpox itself. The would-be revisionist is P. Razzell in *Edward Jenner's Cowpox Vaccine: The History of a Medical Myth,* Sussex: Caliban
Books, 1977, and *The Conquest of Smallpox,* by the same publisher, 1977. The
weaknesses of Razzell's theory are exposed in the review of his books by four scientists from the Center for Disease Control in *Bull. Hist. Med.* 55:273-276, 1981.

Sources on Pasteur are included in the bibliographic commentary following
Chapter 8.

10
SPECIFIC THERAPY

The tracing of Western conceptions of disease would not be complete without a survey of therapy. In part this is because disease concepts tend to dictate approaches to treatment. If you believe in the germ theory of disease, your efforts are directed toward killing the invading bacteria. If you believe rheumatoid arthritis results from an inflammation of the linings of the joints, you give the sufferer anti-inflammatory agents such as aspirin and corticosteroids.

But there is another aspect to the relationship between therapy and concepts of disease which is less often considered. Many times over the centuries, therapy has helped shape concepts of disease. In the seventeenth century the observation that cinchona was efficacious in only one type of fever gave impetus to the idea that there were such things as specific diseases. In the late nineteenth century the treatment of certain endocrine conditions, notably myxedema (hypothyroidism), pointed to the notion that disease could result from a lack or absence of substances, now termed hormones.

This concept received accelerated acceptance as a result of work on beriberi, a crippling, even fatal, disease caused by a lack of one of the B vitamins. In the zealous phase of early bacteriology previously described, efforts were made in the Dutch

East Indies to identify a specific bacterium as the cause of beri-beri. In the 1890s a disease resembling beriberi fortuitously appeared in chickens near the laboratory in Java where a Dutch commission had set up to study the disease. The chickens were placed under observation, but no causative germs could be isolated. Then, without explanation, the chickens recovered. Suspecting that changes in the chickens' diet may have been responsible, the scientists constructed experiments which led to the conclusion that the disease resulted when the chickens were fed only polished rice. Feeding unpolished rice could reverse the disease process. Here, then, was a disease clearly caused not by the presence of something, but by its absence. From this developed the search for other such substances (they were named vitamins); a new category of diseases had grown out of therapeutic experiments.

Prevention is the medical ideal, but in medicine ideals are rarely realized. For certain diseases, cancer for example, no preventive is known. For others, such as venereal diseases, the mere availability of effective preventive measures has not eliminated the need for treatment. A good deal of human suffering results from accidents and assaults, categories that are considered diseases only in special psychological circumstances. Given the human condition as it exists, it is unlikely that medicine will ever be completely preventive. The need for cure has always been with us and always will be.

The two basic approaches to therapy are drugs and surgery. Other forms, such as nursing, psychotherapy, radiation, and physical therapy, despite their real importance, are omitted from what follows because of limitations of space. Also beyond the scope of this chapter is that ancient and enduring species of treatment known as quackery. Omitting quackery is historically questionable, because the distinction between legitimate physician and quack can not always be made on the basis of scientific ignorance or efficacy of treatment. By these criteria all earlier physicians who practiced heroic therapy – bleeding, vomiting, purging – could be labeled quacks. But such a conclusion does not survive closer scrutiny. Physicians have always functioned in a state of relative ignorance. Quackery involves moral considerations as well: willful ignorance or the knowledge that the proffered therapy will not do what is claimed for it. As such, it is beyond the scope of this chapter.

Another form of therapy is folk medicine, a story as old and uninterrupted as that of quackery. Elements of folk medicine will appear in the discussion of empiricism that follows, but in any definitive sense it, too, is beyond our present aim.

Limiting our domain to therapy by drugs and surgery still leaves a formidable historical task. Four thousand years of therapeutics have seen too many medicines and operations and too many notions of why a given intervention worked to be explored in detail here. Instead we shall look only briefly on the tapestry as a whole, then consider in somewhat more detail how simple trial-and-error therapeutics slowly evolved into the more scientific approach of today.

The Philosophy of Therapy

For anyone who has not paused to ponder the matter, the philosophy of therapy might appear to be a rather straightforward matter. Knowing the nature of the disease he has diagnosed, the physician utilizes the best available method to restore normal physiological processes. Gangrene has set in – cut off the afflicted part. Pneumonia has produced a plethora of blood in the lungs – open a vein and restore the balance. In practice, however, the physician's philosophy of treatment has rarely been so uncomplicated. His motives for intervening and the methods employed almost always were shaped by a complex interplay of psychological and cultural forces, which at times he himself could not appreciate.

The complexity of motivation in therapy can be seen in the categories of forces shaping the treatment of syphilis before the twentieth century. The first was empirical knowledge, the physician's understanding of the mechanism of the disease and the curative powers and toxicity of his remedy. As Paracelsus reportedly put it, "the physician must be exactly acquainted with the illness before he can know with what medicine to conquer it."[1] One problem here is that in terms of causation, as we have seen, physicians were not "exactly acquainted" with any important human disease until a century or so ago. This ignorance was partially ameliorated by the fact that understanding causation is

not always needed to effect a cure, as the many successful treatments of cancer now attest. At times, on purely empirical
grounds, physicians have derived therapies that must be considered specific by any reasonable use of the term.

Theorization also shapes the nature of therapeutics, even
when the prevailing theory is later shown to have been factually
bereft. This is exemplified in the first decision the physician
faces in a therapeutic situation – to be active or conservative.
Here much depends on the physician's theoretical confidence in
the healing power of nature. The Hippocratics placed great
emphasis on assisting nature and gave to medicine the concept of
primum non nocere (above all do no harm). Later, in Rome,
Asclepiades would ridicule the "expectant therapy" of the Hippocratics as the "contemplation of death." Thus the essential decision in treatment – to intervene or not – is as old as the profession
itself.

It was theory based on analogy that produced the doctrine of
signatures which helped direct therapeutics in the sixteenth century. It was argued that God had provided a remedy for every
disease and that the only problem was finding it. The answer
was found in the nature of the plants employed. Saffron, because
it was yellow, would cure jaundice. Kidney-shaped leaves were
used against renal disease, and so on. Though religious and
philosophical in origins, the doctrine of signatures accumulated
a large body of empirical evidence that appeared to support
physicians who espoused it. Its fatal shortcoming lay in its first
principles, its a priori reasoning. As it turned out, God simply
was not working His mysterious ways by leaving His signature
on all the medicinal plants.

Economic and other social forces can influence the philosophy
of therapeutics. Lady Mary Montagu anticipated fiscal opposition from the medical profession to her plans to introduce smallpox inoculation into England, writing from Constantinople in
1716 that she "should not fail to write to some of our doctors very
particularly about it, if I knew any one of them that I thought
had virtue enough to destroy such a considerable branch of their
revenue for the good of mankind."[2] A current example of economics and therapy is the widespread use of vitamin B_{12}. Vitamin B_{12} deficiency is a rare condition in the United States, yet
the number of persons receiving regular injections of the vitamin

must run in the thousands. Some of this might be justified on grounds of placebo effect, but economic considerations are almost certainly at play as well.

Another example of cultural effects on medical treatment is seen in the treatment extended King Louis XIV when he was ill, perhaps with typhoid fever. In the year before the episode in question, the mineral antimony had fallen into general disrepute as a therapeutic agent. After Louis was treated and recovered (in spite of, rather than because of, the antimony), the mineral returned to widespread favor in the form of tartar emetic. Emulating our leaders is not limited to matters of fashion. Besides putting men in narrow ties and button-down collars, John Kennedy put a host of persons with back pain into therapeutic rocking chairs.

Even religious and moral considerations have shaped the history of therapy. In part it was moral distinctions in the Renaissance that kept the lower classes under the punishing influence of mercury in the treatment of syphilis while the upper classes shifted to the more benign, but equally inefficacious, guaiacum. Physicians are of course still subject to such moral judgments. In the 1940s and 1950s, before alcoholism became a disease, it was not unknown to punish drunks in the emergency room with injections of paraldehyde, a particularly painful sedative when placed intramuscularly. The punishment was augmented by dividing the dose in two, so that both buttocks were made to atone.

A final category must be added to our general considerations, and that is the poorly understood need for treatment which so many persons exhibit. Sir William Osler (1849–1919) once said that the "desire to take medicine is, perhaps, the greatest feature which distinguishes man from other animals."[3] It is, of course, an imperfect distinction, since a number of animals engage in self-medication, raising the possibility that the behavior is at least partly determined by genes. It has been speculated that human beings developed similar instinctive behavior, in the selection of foods for health and of certain plants to combat illness. At the moment it is impossible to sort out cultural and genetic influences in the compulsion for medication manifested by so many persons. It is nonetheless certain that pressure from patients has had much to do with patterns of therapy in history. In the second century Galen was convinced the public wanted more, not fewer, drugs and that if the therapy was novel, so much the better.

Nor is the patients' willingness to expose themselves to dangerous treatments limited to swallowing new nostrums. In the preface to *The Doctor's Dilemma*, G. B. Shaw described a type known to all surgeons when he wrote:

There are men and women whom the operating table seems to fascinate: half-alive people who through vanity, or hypochondria, or a craving to be the constant objects of anxious attention or what not, lose such feeble sense as they ever had of the value of their own organs and limbs. They seem to care as little for mutilation as lobsters or lizards, which at least have the excuse that they grow new claws and new tails if they lose the old ones.[4]

The forces governing the selection of the drug therapy and of surgical procedures have not been simply the nature of the affliction and the probability that the therapeutic intervention would be efficacious in strictly medical terms. Indeed, at times elements we would identify as scientific have been of only minor importance. Other determinants have included physicians' belief in occult powers, religious forces in general, philosophical and other theorization, economics, cultural influences including faddism, and the willingness, approaching a psychological imperative, to try the new which has characterized both physicians and patients over the years.

Survey of Medical Therapy

We have already learned something of therapy before the Greeks, the mixture of religion and magic that characterized primitive medicine as well as that of the Egyptians and Assyrians. The Hippocratics, with their relative indifference to the notion of specific diseases, were not likely to emphasize specific therapy. They tailored their curative approach to the individual patient and relied on a general regimen including diet in the modern sense. The use of drugs was minimal. The Dogmatists, later followers of the Hippocratic approach, made two important contributions to the evaluation of therapy: experiences, they taught, if they are to be of value, must be repeated many times,

and negative tests must be reported as well as those which suc-
ceed. Had these two principles been followed with anything like
fidelity, later physicians might have escaped a good deal of the
chaos that came to characterize medical therapy. But the
wisdom of the Dogmatists would not be rediscovered until most
of the nineteenth century had passed.

Ancient Rome witnessed the recurring confrontation that has
marked the history of therapy: conservatism versus activism,
rationalism versus experience, the moderation of the regimen
versus polypharmacy and bloodletting. In the first century B.C.
Asclepiades limited sharply the number of drugs he employed,
greatly softened the application of bloodletting and purgatives,
and returned to many of the modalities that had characterized
the Hippocratic regimen. For a while he, and the Methodists
who followed him, held sway. But just as in the matter of disease
causation, the therapy that dominated European thinking for
some 1500 years after Rome was the therapy of Galen developed
in the second century. This, as noted, meant bleeding, purging,
and polypharmacy. For Galen, the more remedies in a prescription the better. Given a wide array of medicinals, the wisdom of
the body would select the appropriate drugs. It was this principle that would be hurled again and again in the faces of those
who tried to adopt the notion of specificity in treatment, the
principle of the "bad cobbler who tries to fit everybody with the
same shoe."[5] Polypharmacy was Galen's legacy, and it dominated
later therapy the way his humoralism dominated ideas of pathology. In the seventeenth century Sydenham's famous Venice
treacle had sixty-five ingredients and his theriac, seventy-two. In
Galenic therapeutics, then, we find the strange and fundamental
contradiction which can be detected in prescribing practices
even today, a heavy reliance on drugs and surgery, along with a
belief in the healing powers of nature.

The pharmacologic Bible underpinning Galenic therapeutics
was the *Materia medica* compiled by Dioscorides (fl. A.D. 50–70).
As a military surgeon under Nero in the last half of the first century A.D., Dioscorides had ample opportunity to become acquainted with the plants of the Mediterranean. Using taste and
smell as his main criteria of therapeutic efficacy, he identified
some 950 medicinal agents, among them 600 plant, 80 animal,

and 50 mineral. Testimony to the enduring influence of Dioscorides is found in the German pharmacopoeia of 1910, which still contained 90 drugs from his original five books.

In Dioscorides we find the seeds of another concept that has marked the history of therapeutics, the use of a drug as both specific and panacea. The search for a panacea is as old as, and may be associated with, the quest for immortality. For Galen and his followers in the Middle Ages it was "that hellish brew," theriac. For Renaissance physicians after Paracelsus, it was mineral therapy, in particular antimony. Drugs that were found efficacious in one medical condition were quickly applied to situations in which they were useless. Digitalis alleviated dropsy and so was tried in tuberculosis, pneumonia, typhoid fever, and mental illness. Iodine cured goiter and became a panacea for cancer, skin diseases, heart disease, epilepsy, tuberculosis, malaria, cholera, and arteriosclerosis.

During the Middle Ages and Renaissance, Galenic therapy was enriched by what might be called pharmacologic exorcism. The phenomenon was based in part on a return to the notion that disease was demonic in nature. To drive the evil spirits from the body, disgusting remedies were concocted which to this day remain a monument to human ingenuity. As Montaigne put it, "For them everything which was not in ordinary use took the place of drugs." John Hall, a physician and William Shakespeare's son-in-law, who died in 1635, prescribed among other things webs of spiders, animal excreta, and dried cocks' windpipes, and in one of his own illnesses he had a live pigeon opened and applied to the soles of his feet to "draw down the vapors."[6]

All of this seems a far cry from the ordered regimens of the Hippocratics and Galen, and so it was. By the time of John Hall the therapeutic situation had become hopeless, a development that dates to the sixteenth century and the beginning of four hundred years of chaos in therapy. The search for specificity in diseases and remedies initiated by Paracelsus in the same century was not the movement that would direct the future. Galenic traditionalism remained. The importance of exotic drugs was recognized, and there was a revival of Hippocratism with its implicit nonspecificity. It was a milieu that overpowered the best minds of the time. Vesalius, perhaps the greatest medical innovator of the Renaissance, could manage little change in the prevailing therapy. Nor could the most original medical thinkers in the three hundred years that followed, regardless of their rigorous dedication to science in other aspects of medicine.

In the ideological struggle that began in the sixteenth century, the Galenists relied heavily, though not exclusively, on vegetable compounds, whereas the Paracelsians put their major reliance on minerals. By the beginning of the eighteenth century the dispute was largely resolved, and neither party could claim a lasting victory. The Galenists were gone; few Paracelsians could be identified; and in their wake came a concerned effort to purge all worthless drugs from the pharmacopoeia. This latter process reveals again the influence of nonmedical thought on medical practices. The Enlightenment tended to reject notions of magic. Because they had at times been associated with magical uses, a number of useful drugs were thrown out with the bathwater, including opium, quinine, iron, mercury, and belladonna. At the same time a number of efficacious remedies were added, a few of which are described below. For purposes of this survey a single observation can be made: no matter what changes occurred in medical thinking about the nature of disease, the basic approach to treatment remained largely the same. Thus, astounding though it seems, treatment aimed at restoring humoral balance was still a principal part of therapy through the first half of the nineteenth century.

Three Forms of Empiricism

After this brief Baedeker on the history of medical therapy, it remains to examine the matter from another point of view. In a very real sense all therapy is empirical. Even if a drug's mechanism of action is fully understood and the physician has wide experience with it, when it is given to a patient for the first time, it is an empirical act. The medication may work precisely as expected, or the patient may suffer an idiosyncratic, and therefore unpredictable, reaction. Ultimately the matter can be resolved only by trial and error. In the development of new therapies, however, there are levels of empiricism, degrees of methodological sophistication, which tend to determine the likelihood that a given drug trial will yield valid results. For our purposes these will be termed crude, refined, and controlled empiricism, listed in the order of their historical development.

Crude Empiricism

Easily the most debilitating mental process in the evolution of medical therapy has been the fallacy *post hoc ergo propter hoc* (after which, therefore because of which). This is the logical lapse that causes one to conclude that the lightning which struck a nearby tree during the last month of pregnancy has produced a disfiguring birthmark on the child. Or that recovery from pneumonia is due to the vigorous bloodletting employed. Or that a winter without a cold proves the efficacy of Vitamin C. The phenomenon's pervasiveness, historically and at present, among the learned and others, is so thoroughgoing that one is tempted to label it an inborn error of the human intellect. In terms of therapy, *post hoc, propter hoc* translates to the proposition that the disappearance of symptoms is equivalent to a medical cure of the disease. The fallacy makes no allowance for the fact that many diseases have spontaneous but temporary remissions, and that most are self-limited. Long-range thinking came to medical science only relatively recently and has not reached all physicians even today.

Crude empiricism, of course, cannot escape *post hoc, propter hoc* and indeed relies on such reasoning for its validation. It is anecdotal by nature, and at times a single anecdote may be all that is required to sanctify a given remedy, at least in one physician's mind. The remedy is applied; if the symptoms disappear within a reasonable length of time, the remedy worked, and it will be employed again the next time a similar set of symptoms appears.

Despite its innate weaknesses, crude empiricism produced a number of remedies which, by present standards, could do what they were believed to do. Several such drugs might even be labeled as specifics, mercury to promote the excretion of bodily fluids, for example, and the bark of the cinchona tree in the treatment of malaria. Another example is opium, whose earliest use in the control of pain cannot be dated. Like many substances that found their way into medical practice, opium probably derived from folk medicine. We know it was used by healers in ancient Egypt and Greece and freely employed by the Alexandrian empiricists. Its addictive qualities were all too well known to Marcus Aurelius after his exposure to Galen's "theriac of Demetrios." Opium was such a favorite remedy with Sydenham that he was called, we are told, "Opiophilos." At least one contemporary could not agree with Sydenham's free use of the poppy because, as the critics said, "it reduces men to an Estate more like that of death than life." It was frequently prescribed by Boerhaave, the most famous clinician of the eighteenth century, and along with alcohol comprised the "charm" that probably accounted for part of the success of John Brown's system of medicine later in the same century. The active ingredient, morphine, was isolated in 1806 in what is recognized as the first significant contribution of chemistry to pharmacology.

The discovery and persistence of opium is not surprising. Pain is part of the human condition, and contrary to some moral preachments, prolonged severe pain is not ordinarily an ennobling experience. In medicine generally, and surgery before the advent of general anesthesia, opium was queen of the anodynes. As Oliver Wendell Holmes remarked, "opium . . . the Creator himself seems to prescribe, for we often see the scarlet poppy growing in the cornfields, as if it were foreseen that wherever there is hunger to be fed there must also be pain to be soothed."[7]

Heroic Therapy

Historically the more important feature of crude empiricism has been generation of therapeutic excesses. If a little of a drug appears to work, the temptation is to try a bit more, to match the severity of the disease with even more severe therapy. Uncontrolled empiricism did not have to lead to excesses – homeopaths achieved wide popularity in the nineteenth century using infinitesimal doses – but the danger of abuse was always there and, all too often, there to see. The single most persistent therapeutic modality in the history of disease has been bloodletting, and the excesses to which it was carried at times require a discussion of the rationale behind it.

Over the centuries three principal ideas contributed to the

theoretical basis for bloodletting. The first was Galen's example of the needle prick. We now understand that infection determines whether a pricked finger heals cleanly or results in an inflamed, swollen (plethoric) condition. For Galen if a pricked finger became inflamed it was because the body itself was plethoric, that is, full of unevacuated waste products. Bleeding, by relieving the plethora, would permit healing to occur.

The second conceptual foundation of bloodletting was the doctrine of laudable wound hemorrhage. Earlier we encountered the doctrine of laudable pus, the notion that pus resulted from a process that was requisite to healing. Hippocratic physicians came to believe that the complications of wounds, pus and inflammation, were due to the blood and not to the object producing the wound. A reasonable amount of hemorrhage, then, was not an undesirable situation but one that promoted healing by drying the wound.

The final and most influential theoretical basis was the doctrine of physiologic excess, the imbalance already discussed in treating the notion of humoral pathology. There are numerous disease states in which the symptoms and signs strongly suggest excess. In fever the skin is hot, the face flushed, the pulse rapid, the thought hectic. In dropsy the legs and even the abdominal and thoracic cavities are filled with fluid. Inflammation is marked by swelling, pain, redness, and heat, as in a boil. These are common medical conditions, and all are marked by apparent excess: fluid, heat, rapid heart rate, swelling, plethora. For such conditions, the physical findings alone would suggest a definite rationality for the process of taking blood.

Public acceptance of bloodletting became as entrenched as that of the profession, so much so that physicians who tried to limit the use of the lancet ran into the same pressures facing the modern physician who is reluctant to prescribe penicillin for the common cold. The faith was still being kept in the nineteenth century. On the death of Byron the London *Times* reportedly had this to say: "Lord Byron died in consequence of refusing to be bled when he had an inflammation of the chest. When it was proposed to him to be bled, he answered that he would not, for more people died, he believed, by the lancet than the lance."[8]

The history of bloodletting has been practically uninterrupted.

It is true that there is no mention of bleeding in the Ebers Papyrus, but it was used by the Hippocratics, who looked on bleeding as equivalent to reducing dietary intake. That they were moderates in this aspect of therapy is probably reflected by the fact that there are few references to bloodletting in Hippocratic writings and no specific work on the subject. It was bloodletting that separated the two greatest medical figures of Hellenic Alexandria. Herophilus, as a humoralist, relied on drugs and bleeding, while Erasistratus, as a solidist, opposed heavy bleeding in favor of diet. After Galen, as with so many other aspects of medicine, the emphasis on bloodletting was established for centuries to come.

Following Galen's example, most of the great figures in medical history, regardless of their other contributions, remained true to the lance. They all bled – Avicenna, Arnold of Villanova, Fracastoro (albeit conservatively), Paracelsus, Sydenham to excess, Baglivi, Harvey, and in the eighteenth century Benjamin Rush, Cullen, Stahl, Hoffmann, and Boerhaave. Despite the rise of therapeutic skepticism, Broussais's influence led France in 1833 to import some 42 million leeches for medicinal purposes.

In the nineteenth century and earlier, venesection had been joined by other evacuant methods, which together constitute what is called heroic therapy. The principal cathartic in terms of abuse was calomel or mercurous chloride. The doses employed were designed more to move mountains than bowels. In 1844 an American physician, perhaps hyperbolically, indicated that it was not rare to use *"table spoon doses every hour,* until the patient held, somewhere between the mouth and the rectum, a *pound* of the article."[9] The *United States Dispensatory* of 1858 listed the purgative doses as 5 to 15 grains, while by the 1940s the maximum recommended dose was only 2 grains. The tablespoon dose mentioned above would contain some 250 grains.

Excesses, some all but incredible, marked bloodletting as well. Within one year Louis XIII was bled 47 times, purged on 215 occasions, and received 212 clysters (a medicinal enema). During the last four years of her life the physician Rasori (1766–1837) bled a thirty-one-year-old woman 1,309 times or, for practical purposes, daily. During his short terminal illness George Washington was treated with calomel, emetic tartar, vapors of vinegar, blisters on his extremities and throat, and venesections totaling an estimated ninety ounces, or almost half the blood volume of an average adult male. It is not surprising, perhaps, that reportedly one of his last articulated desires was a request that he be allowed to die without further medical assistance.

By 1860 the worst features of heroic therapy were disappearing in the United States and England. Interestingly, bloodletting diminished without much literary interchange among members of the medical profession. The reasons for its demise were concocted largely after the fact. Diseases had changed, it was said, and thus bleeding was no longer appropriate. Or the population was debilitated from the effects of industrialization and was thereby no longer a candidate for heroic therapy.

In part also the disaffection with bloodletting came from the first application of controls to what had heretofore been ordinary crude empiricism. This came in 1835 at the hands of a member of the Paris Clinical School, Pierre-Charles-Alexandre Louis (1787–1872). Before Louis, François Magendie, the French clinician and experimentalist, had abandoned bleeding in pneumonia only to learn how completely ingrained the practice was – his interns continued to bleed patients behind his back. Magendie is also credited with placing pharmacology on a scientific basis, therefore opening up a new era of experimental pharmacology, with his work on strychnine, emetine, quinine, iodine, and bromine. In the process he effectively prevented Parisian physicians from embracing total therapeutic nihilism, as they might have done after Louis's exploitation of what came to be called the numerical method.

Louis's accomplishment, succinctly put, was the application of statistics to clinical medicine. His aim was to determine the effect of bloodletting on the duration of illness and mortality rate of pneumonia, which thanks to Corvisart and Laennec could now be diagnosed with reasonable accuracy. Louis did not attempt a controlled study in the current sense, that is, by bleeding some patients and not others. Rather, he sought to demonstrate the effects of timing and the amount of blood withdrawn on the course of the illness. By later statistical standards his study was flawed and certain of his conclusions were improper, but his solid common sense overcame the deficiencies of his method.

It should be emphasized that Louis did not advocate total abandonment of bloodletting in inflammatory diseases. But his reservations and, most importantly, his use of statistics in reaching his conclusions, infused the antiheroic movement with the one element that had always been missing—a scientific method for testing the anecdotal nature of crude empiricism. The ensuing skepticism spread to many students who worked in the Parisian center of clinical training in the first half of the nineteenth century, including a number of Americans. One of these, Oliver Wendell Holmes, would later utter what is easily the most quoted assessment of the state of therapeutics around 1860. "Throw out opium . . . a few specifics which our art did not discover . . . wine . . . and the vapors which produce the miracle of anesthesia, and I firmly believe that if the whole materia medica, *as now used,* could be sunk to the bottom of the sea, it would be all the better for mankind—and all the worse for the fishes."[10]

The demise of heroic therapy, insofar as it has died, began in the United States around 1825. Though precision is difficult in such matters, it is likely that public disaffection with heroic medicine had more to do with its decline than judgments within the medical profession itself. The rise of medical sects coincided with the decline in popularity of heroic therapy. As the public became increasingly disaffected with bleeding, it abandoned regular physicians and turned to homeopaths, naturopaths, hydropaths, herbalists, Thomsonians, and the many other sects that preached a greater role for nature in healing. It appears, then, that heroic therapy was abandoned by the medical profession only after the regular practitioner and his therapy were in the process of abandonment by the public.

Refined Empiricism

To consider an example of refined empiricism we must return to the eighteenth century and William Withering (1741-1799), who graduated from Edinburgh University in 1766 and finally entered practice in Birmingham, England. For some time thereafter he made a habit of returning the thirty miles to see patients in Stafford, where he had first practiced. On one occasion, while waiting for the horses to be changed, he was asked to see a woman with dropsy. He concluded that her prognosis was grim, and thus, a few weeks later, was surprised to find her much improved. His patient attributed her remarkable recovery to a herbal tea she had been given by an old woman of Shropshire, who had long kept her remedy a secret. As a proficient, self-trained botanist, Withering rather quickly concluded that of the twenty or so herbs making up the concoction, the active ingredient had to be foxglove, or digitalis as we would call it. His conviction led him to ten years of experimenting with foxglove in the treatment of dropsy. In the process he discovered that the dropsical tissues could be unburdened of their fluid without the toxic doses used by his lay colleague. Vomiting and diarrhea were not needed; instead any one of a number of events indicated proper dosage – slowing of the pulse, increased urinary output, nausea, or mild diarrhea.

In 1785, at five shillings a copy, Withering published *An Account of the Foxglove, etc.*, in which he reported 170 cases of his own in addition to the experience of fourteen colleagues. What had he done that justifies the use of the term refined empiricism? He had experimented on animals as well as human beings. He had meticulously recorded the findings in a large number of cases before announcing his conclusions. He had published his failures as well as his successes, thus attempting, unsuccessfully as it turned out, to counteract the panacea effect. And he had demonstrated that even after empiricism proves a remedy to be successful, it will be used to better effect if something is learned of its mode of action. The old lady had intoxicated her patients in order to cure. Withering attained the same happy end using smaller, properly timed doses, because he recognized that digitalis produced its effects by acting on the heart and kidneys.

Controlled Empiricism

To this point the implicit message has been that empiricism, in its earlier form, was not a very efficient way to evaluate new therapy. The unresolved problem, to reiterate, was to be certain that the drug effected the observed improvement. In certain circumstances the nature of the disease might have obviated this difficulty. Historically, diseases such as rabies and tuberculous meningitis were uniformly fatal. Had someone developed a treatment which cured two successive cases of rabies, important conclusions could have been drawn despite the smaller number of cases and absence of controls. Such exceptions prove no general case. The psychological and physiological response of human beings to medication is so perversely complex that *post hoc, propter hoc* will always cast its dubious shadow on uncontrolled clinical experimentation. In a vague way, the problem of cause and effect must have been appreciated by many investigators over the years. As early as the second century we find Galen attempting to control a therapeutic test by comparing different agents in the same situation. To demonstrate the superiority of vinegar in alleviating burns by thapsia, he annointed several locations with the irritant substance, then treated the sites variously with vinegar, water, olive oil, oil of rose, and so on.

Still, over the years, we find few examples of the quest for control in therapeutic investigations. The next example of note is that of the Scottish naval surgeon James Lind (1716–1794) and his work with scurvy. Lind lived in the eighteenth century, and thus it is moderately surprising to find that the curative effect of citrus fruits on scurvy was widely known in the sixteenth and seventeenth centuries. Indeed, before Lind, a successful controlled study of sorts had been carried out by the East India Company in 1600. On the first expedition to India, one of the four sailing vessels was provided with lemon juice. The sailors on the chosen ship remained almost completely free of scurvy, whereas those on the other three ships were hard hit. Why then was such evidence effectively ignored by the British Admiralty for almost two hundred years? The principal explanation appears to be that the phenomenon of the voyage to India could not be consistently reproduced. This was because the scurvy of earlier times rarely existed as a pure disease. Sailors and others who had insufficient access to sources of vitamin C developed scurvy, but they also suffered multiple nutritional diseases, perhaps complicated by bacterial infections. In such syndromes, fruit juice alone could not be expected to produce a uniform cure.

Lind described his experiment as follows:

On 20 May 1747, I took twelve patients in the scurvy, on board the *Salisbury* at sea. Their cases were as similar as I could have them. They all in

general had putrid gums, the spots and lassitude, with weakness of their
knees. They lay together in one place . . . and had one diet common to
all. . . . Two of these were ordered each a quart of cider a day. Two
others took twenty-five gutts [drops] of elixir vitriol three times a
day. . . . Two others took two spoonfuls of vinegar three times a
day. . . . Two of the worst patients . . . were put under a course of sea-
water. . . . Two others had each two oranges and one lemon. . . . They
continued but six days under this course, having consumed the quantity
that could be spared. . . . The two remaining patients took [a complicated prescription]. . . . The consequence was, that the most sudden and
visible good effects were perceived from the use of the oranges and
lemons.[11]

But the force of such results had nothing like that which would
accrue to them today. Lind himself continued to believe that
"moist sea air" was equally important in causing scurvy, and that
a change in air was a first requirement in treating the disease.
The British Admiralty did not adopt Lind's regimen until 1795,
but this must not be looked upon merely as an example of bureaucratic myopia. Other reasons were involved. Citrus fruits
were expensive and difficult to preserve. Some authorities held
that sauerkraut worked equally well. And finally, the West In-
dian limes that were adopted for economic reasons were deficient in the critical vitamin, with the result that as late as 1875
scurvy reportedly occurred among sailors taking lime juice in
the prescribed amounts. The work of Withering and Lind did not
establish a new form of therapeutic investigation, but their innovations indicated the lines along which controlled empiricism
would develop.

Paul Ehrlich and the Magic Bullet

Despite a few early attempts, a systematic approach to developing and testing new drugs did not mature and produce practical results until near the beginning of the twentieth century.
When it arrived it was thoroughly enmeshed in the new bacteriology. Once germs were identified causally with human disease,
it was only natural to seek agents for their destruction, a quest
that was by no means new. Fracastoro in the sixteenth century

advocated chilling and heating the patient, evacuation, blood-letting, and the administration of antipathetic agents. Even specificity was conceived and advocated. Around 1714 a physician suggested that a specific drug might be used to attack a given infection by the "little worms" which these early microscopists had identified with disease. But such speculations, as we have seen, can be discovered in the history of all the major concepts of disease. Their value is realized only when they are exploited in ways that finally succor ailing human beings. This aspect of the story is rooted in an endeavor apparently unrelated to the struggle against disease – the industrial development of artificial dyes.

When he synthesized aniline purple or mauve in 1856, while yet but eighteen years of age, William Henry Perkin (1838-1907) initiated what would become a revolution in the dye industry. As more and better synthetic dyes became available, they began attracting the attention of medical scientists, the most important of whom for our purposes was Carl Weigert of Breslau (1845-1904). Between 1870 and 1880 Weigert perfected techniques of superimposed staining which provided contrast between cells of different types and made easier the identification of bacteria in tissues. In so doing he helped establish the fact that would be crucial to the development of chemotherapy: different cells have affinities for different stains.

Weigert imparted his techniques and knowledge of staining to a cousin, the Silesian Paul Ehrlich (1854-1915), who as a lad had already experimented with dyeing live flowers and animals. The basis of what would become chemotherapy was Ehrlich's deduction, almost childishly simple to the modern mind, that altering a chemical's structure, even subtly, would alter its effects. At a critical juncture chance once again entered the picture. Ehrlich came across a work in which the author maintained that the question of lead poisoning could be resolved by placing slices of liver, heart, and kidney tissues in a solution of lead and measuring the amount of lead absorbed by each tissue over time.

In this revelatory conception Ehrlich was back to the phenomenon that focussed his major scientific contributions, the affinity between tissues and chemicals. The next step led to his work with specificity in therapy. Was it possible that bacteria might have an affinity for chemicals that would prove lethal to the germs but harmless to surrounding cells, that might serve as "charmed bullets," as he would call them later? Ehrlich's "magic bullet" would prove to be a chimera, but the ideal sustained his efforts at the time. After some success using trypan red against trypanosomal parasites, he turned his attention to syphilis, at that time a far more important disease in nontropical countries.

For his chemical Ehrlich chose an organic arsenical, in part because arsenic had been shown to have a specific effect on the trypanosome that produced African sleeping sickness. In 1909 he was joined by the Japanese Sahachiro Hata (1873–1938), who had managed to induce syphilis in rabbits, thus providing Ehrlich with the necessary experimental model. In a paradigm of thoroughness and persistence, the investigators manipulated their arsenical compound 605 times in search of a drug that would meet Ehrlich's principles. The 606th effort in 1909 produced arsphenamine (salvarsan), whose toxicity was within acceptable limits. Neoarsphenamine, or 912, was derived three years later and proved even more satisfactory.

The work of Ehrlich did not fully satisfy the principles with which he had embarked. His hope for a single killing dose was not realized; periodic injections were necessary over a period of months. Still, nothing can detract from the importance of 606 and 912. Salvarsan was announced in 1910, and within a year Ehrlich had distributed 60,000 doses. The reactions of clinicians need not be imagined; one was recorded by a contemporary, who said, "the chancre, the rash, the Wassermann reaction, all cleared up like magic. People . . . were astounded. . . . It was a miracle."[12]

The Sulfonamides

The promise of Ehrlich's method was far greater than its practical application in the treatment of syphilis. One is reminded of the differences between Jenner's limited cowpox model and the method that promised universal application, as exemplified in Pasteur's work with chicken cholera, anthrax, and rabies. Surely Ehrlich's success with arsphenamine could be duplicated for many pathogenic microbes by nothing more than a massive program of chemical manipulation. As it turned out, bacteria and viruses were not as susceptible to chemotherapy as the spirochete of syphilis or the protozoan of sleeping sickness. What followed has been termed the Doldrum Years. Dead end piled on dead end, and by the early 1930s scientists generally had given up on chemotherapy for bacterial diseases.

At this point the story returns to an industry involved in the production of dyes. In 1927 the I. G. Farbenindustrie of Germany took on a medical scientist, Gerhard Domagk (1895–1964), as director of research in experimental pathology and biology. Domagk set about testing the protective action of a group of azo dyes on mice which had been infected with streptococci. In 1932 he discovered that one of the dyes, prontosil, would cure mice after injection of what was ordinarily a lethal dose of the cocci, results that he mysteriously did not publish until three years later.

A team of scientists at the Pasteur Institute then made the surprising discovery that prontosil would not destroy streptococci in the test tube. From that finding they reasoned that prontosil itself was not the lethal agent, but rather some breakdown product that was produced only in the animal's body. Their reasoning proved accurate, and the lethal ingredient, sulfanilamide, was isolated. The work by the French team was of more than academic interest. Prontosil was under patent, but sulfanilamide had been discovered in 1908 and was in the public domain. This meant no monopoly was possible and placed the price of sulfanilamide within reasonable bounds. At this point the story scarcely meets the criteria of scientific altruism, if, as has been postulated, Domagk delayed publication of his prontosil work for over two years because he, too, knew that sulfanilamide was the active portion of the molecule and he was searching for even more effective varieties that could be patented as prontosil had been. For his work Domagk received the 1939 Nobel Prize in medicine and physiology.

In 1938 sulfapyridine was synthesized and found to be at least the equal of sulfanilamide, with one important difference. Sulfapyridine was effective against the pneumococcus as well. Physicians finally had a way to deal with pneumonia, which was known as the "captain of the men of death" because it was the fatal complication in so many other medical conditions. Sulfapyridine was soon replaced by the safer sulfadiazine and it, in turn, largely by sulfasoxazole. Thus, by the time of the Second World War, a number of common contagious diseases were susceptible to a measure of specific therapy.

Penicillin

The world knew nothing about it, but years before the sulfa drugs began to realize their potential, serendipity had once again worked its wondrous way. In 1928 in a small London laboratory, a Scottish physician, Alexander Fleming (1881–1955), discovered that one of his staphylococci cultures had been contaminated by a mold. In keeping with Pasteur's admonition, Fleming's mind was prepared for such chance observations. In contrast with many of his colleagues, for years he had made a practice of keeping his used cultures for two or three weeks to see if anything "interesting" happened. He was further prepared by his earlier work with lysozyme, which had taught him the importance of the contaminant. Thus, instead of throwing out the contaminated culture with an appropriate oath, he decided to pursue the matter further. The first step showed that his unwelcome intruder was a species of the fungus, penicillium.

An important limitation of sulfa drugs is that they are bacteriostatic rather than bactericidal. They work rather slowly by arresting reproduction, thus counting on the body's defenses to overwhelm the invading microbes. The fact that there exist in nature microbes capable of actually killing other germs has been known for a long time. In 1889 the Frenchman J.-A. Villemin claimed credit for naming the phenomenon when he coined the term "antibiosis" for the process in which one living body exerts a destructive effect on another with which it is in close contact. Pasteur apparently was the first to demonstrate antibiosis in the world of microorganisms. He noted that if any of several varieties of germs was inoculated into urine containing anthrax, the anthrax stopped growing and sooner or later died out completely. He found, further, that adding these common bacteria to an anthrax culture before injecting it protected the test animal against the disease of anthrax. With beguiling brevity, he concluded that his observations held genuine promise for therapy.

Fleming's role in the story of penicillin generally has been exaggerated. There is no doubt that he retained a certain low interest in the substance and a conviction that it had therapeutic potential greater than that of the sulfonamides. He demonstrated its low toxicity and used it with some success by applying it locally to wounds. At this point he was hampered by his inability to purify the substance, by his lack of chemical knowledge, and by his inability to find a collaborator with the requisite chemical ability. He was by nature taciturn and lacked the verbal ability and political gifts required at times to translate discovery into application. Beyond all this, there is evidence that he was not convinced that the problem of isolating and purifying the active fraction of penicillium *could* be overcome – as late as 1939 he reportedly advised a colleague to forget penicillin as a potential antibiotic because of its instability.

Credit for purifying penicillin and for overcoming the many problems of mass production belongs to Howard Florey (1898-1968) and his team of Oxford investigators, most notably Ernst Chain (1906-1979), who pointed the group toward penicillin in the first place. Over several years before 1941, these workers produced sufficient amounts of increasingly pure penicillin to demonstrate its protective action on infected animals. Further, it was their efforts at Oxford Hospital that produced the first effective clinical trials. Much of the exaggerated credit which Fleming himself referred to as the "Fleming myth" resulted from the popular and media reaction to the glory heaped on Fleming by Sir Almoth Wright in a letter to the London *Times* on August 31, 1942. Florey consistently refused to be drawn into the ensuing fray. The Nobel committee of 1945 found sufficient merit in all the principals, dividing the award that year among Fleming, Florey, and Chain.

The emphasis of the past few pages has been on the systematic and prospective development of new medicinal chemicals. It remains to say a few final words about the later evolution of clinical experimentation, the continuing effort to eliminate the *post hoc, propter hoc* fallacy from the evaluation of new therapies. The eighteenth-century studies of digitalis by Withering and of citrus fruits by Lind were noteworthy for their exceptionality and not because they were immediately or widely emulated. In the nineteenth century Magendie, Bernard, Pasteur, and others extended the idea of increasingly controlled clinical experimentation to substances of bacteriological and chemical origin. The fact that no dramatically effective drugs emerged from these efforts is more a testimonial to the complexity of the problem than the paucity of the effort. The twentieth century has seen an enormous increase in the number of clinical trials, as well as a steady refinement in their design and major innovations in the application of statistical tests. Out of these efforts have come the blind study (test subject is unaware of the nature of the drug or procedure involved), double-blind (neither investigator nor subject knows), and double-blind cross-over (drug and placebo switched at some point without knowledge of subject or researcher). Since the middle of the twentieth century, then, clinical scientists have had the wherewithal to avoid most of the pitfalls of cause and effect which so consistently trapped their professional progenitors. The larger errors that continue to appear result more from ignorance and misinterpretation than from the methodology itself.

Earlier Surgical Therapy

The role played by surgical thought in the concept of localized disease was discussed in an earlier chapter. Passing mention was made as well of the long split between medicine and surgery, a rift still found in the more or less good-natured bantering between surgeons and internists, such as that attributed to Martin Fischer when he said, "The practice of medicine is a thinker's art, the practice of surgery a plumber's."

The development of the surgery we know is usually pictured as occurring only after the advent of general anesthesia and effective antisepsis. In the late eighteenth century, however, surgeons of the French Academy performed many operations that ordinarily would have been on the historian's list of proscribed procedures. One finds these surgeons treating penetrating abdominal wounds, opening the skull, removing a stone that obstructed the rectum, operating for gallstones and lung abscess, and undertaking cesarian sections.

The absence of effective general anesthesia placed a premium on speed in surgery. William Cheselden in the eighteenth century reportedly removed a bladder stone in fifty-four seconds.

Most major surgery, of course, is not amenable to such feats, and limitations of time further constricted the outlook of earlier operators. The two major obstacles to prolonged intracavitary surgery were not overcome until the nineteenth century was more than half over. Thus the global reach of modern surgery is only a bit over one hundred years of age. In passing, it should be pointed out that the two keys to extending the surgical reach, antisepsis and anesthesia, have been viewed more recently as effects rather than causes of the current enlarged role of surgery. The argument is that as surgery became more important after 1840 (in part due to medicine's decline in public esteem), an interest developed in improved technology as well as surgical technique. Prior to the nineteenth century, however, it is still safe to describe surgery largely as wound surgery.

By the end of the ancient period physicians had all but abandoned the knife. The Arabs, who thought highly of Greek medicine in general, held surgery in low esteem. Well into the Middle Ages, even the better surgeons concerned themselves mainly with dressing wounds and curing ulcers and eschewed operative procedures for hernia, bladder stone, facial disfigurement, and cataract as too dangerous. These operations became the province of itinerant "cutters" and quacks. At this point one frequently encounters historians who maintain that the stasis of surgery in the medieval period was due to an abhorrence of shedding blood, which became institutionalized by the Roman Catholic Church. Strictly speaking, this assessment is no longer tenable. It now seems likely that contemporaries placed differing interpretation on such churchly pronouncements and that, in any event, the practical application of the strictures varied with locale.

Surgery and Paré

The ancient split between medicine and surgery began to be bridged in the late Middle Ages, particularly in Italy. Some of the more prominent surgeons at this time were not only trained in medicine but were clerics as well, and university chairs in anatomy and surgery were joined. The revival of surgery became manifest in the sixteenth century with the work in plastic surgery of Gaspare Tagliacozzi (1545-1599), but most especially with the accomplishments of Ambroise Paré (1510-1590). As with most practicing surgeons of his day, Paré was not an educated man in the humanist tradition. He began as a barber's apprentice, then spent several years as a surgeon in a Paris hospital. His native ability, his understanding of the importance of anatomy, and his wide experience in the great instructor of surgeons, warfare, led Paré to the top of his profession, and his profession to a new respectability. Specifically, he revived the ancient practice of amputating through healthy tissue, thus improving the cure rate in this then common medical situation. He also brought back the ligature, the use of which had been common in Hippocratic times, and reintroduced podalic version, in which a fetus trapped in the uterus is turned so that one or both feet are delivered first. Finally, Paré abandoned the treatment of gunshot wounds (which were thought to be poisoned) with boiling oil, in favor of gentler applications such as turpentine and brandy. Like Paracelsus, Paré wrote in the vernacular, and his works were soon known to English, Dutch, German, and later even Japanese physicians.

John Hunter

No one appeared immediately to exploit Paré's lead. The seventeenth century saw essentially no conceptual or practical advances in the field of surgery. In the eighteenth century, however, another forceful and innovative surgeon appeared, after whom surgery would gradually become an integral and equal partner in the healing arts. John Hunter (1728-1793) was born near Glasgow, which, perhaps significantly, was the only British city that had never separated medicine and surgery. In London under his brother, William (1718-1783), he acquired a passion for anatomy and surgery and then agreed to enroll at Oxford to acquire the needed polish. He was back in London within two months, observing that "they wanted to make an old woman of me, or that I should stuff Latin and Greek at the University; but these schemes I cracked like so many vermin as they came before me."[13] It is likely that missing the usual medical education of the time enhanced rather than penalized Hunter's later career. True, his writings are not as clear and elegant as they might otherwise have been, but neither do they pay much attention to the persistent humoral concepts that narrowed the outlook of many of his contemporaries.

To demonstrate Hunter's main importance, only one of his many contributions will be described here, that being his surgical approach to aneurysm, the condition in which an artery balloons out and at times ruptures. In Hunter's day, surgeons who were daring enough to operate on aneurysms at all, attacked the diseased vessel by ligating immediately above and below the dilated sac, then evacuating the contents. All too often the artery deteriorated, the ligature failed, and a fatal hemorrhage ensued. Hunter instead placed only one ligature, this far up in the direction of the heart where the arterial tissue was completely healthy. He did nothing with the aneurysm itself, which, deprived of the force of the blood pressure, gradually subsided in size.

The new method proved far more efficacious than the old, but it is not Hunter's results that interest us so much as the process that led him to try his operation in the first place. One reason his colleagues ligated close to the aneurysm was their fear that a higher tie would deprive the limb of so much blood that gangrene would result. Hunter was convinced that there were enough smaller arterial branches that he could ligate even the femoral artery, the main vessel supplying the leg, and still avoid gangrene. He had arrived at this conclusion not merely by rationalization, but by experimentation as well, and therein lies the point of recounting the episode. To test his thesis Hunter tied the external carotid artery supplying a half-grown antler of a deer and noted the immediate and apparently dangerous coldness that resulted. Within a week, however, the antler was warm and growth had resumed, because smaller vessels had enlarged and proliferated to take over the function of the destroyed main artery. It was this experimental demonstration of the development of what is called collateral circulation that convinced Hunter his radical departure would work in arterial aneurysms in human beings. His significance, then, is that he demonstrated to surgeons the value of experimentation and physiological understanding. No longer should surgery be based purely on crude empiricism.

Anesthesia

The professional and social status of surgeons was largely repaired by the middle of the nineteenth century, but they still confronted the ancient barriers of pain and infection. Lister's success in dealing with the latter has been related, and it remains to consider the development of anesthesia.

The ordeal of surgery before the development of general anesthesia has been described on many occasions. One of the best is the fictional account based in fact in *Rab and His Friends*, by the Scottish physician John Brown (1810–1882). In the story a woman named Ailie undergoes a total breast amputation with no premedication or anesthesia. In the words of the medical student narrator, she

stepped up on a seat, and laid herself on the table, as her friend the surgeon told her; arranged herself, gave a rapid look at [her husband], shut her eyes, rested herself on me, and took my hand. The operation was at once begun; it was necessarily slow; and chloroform – one of God's best gifts to his suffering children – was then unknown. The surgeon did his work. The pale face showed its pain, but was still and silent. . . . It is over: she is dressed, steps gently and decently down from the table, . . . then, turning to the surgeon and the students, she curtsies, – and in a low, clear voice, begs their pardon if she has behaved ill. The students – all of us – wept like children.[14]

Drugs had been used to reduce the pain of surgery for millennia, probably back into the prehistoric period. All had drawbacks. Some, such as belladonna, simply were not sufficiently anesthetic. Others, opium and alcohol, could produce reasonable anesthesia only with life-threatening doses. A truly efficacious anesthetic not only has to eliminate pain but, for abdominal operations, must produce a deep relaxation of the musculature to allow the retraction the surgeon requires to visualize the operative field. And of course it must be reasonably safe. This combination of features did not come together in one agent until ether was tested in America in the 1840s.

Ether was discovered some three hundred years before our present story begins, and it may even be that Paracelsus knew of its anesthetic properties. In the first half of the nineteenth century, both ether and nitrous oxide were used in a social setting in what were called "ether frolics." It was in this setting that the idea of using it in surgery probably first occurred to Crawford W. Long (1815-1878), a physician in a rural village of Georgia. Long first used ether in 1842 by dropping it on a towel on the patient's face during an operation to remove a tumor on the back of the neck. He repeated his feat in a few other cases, told several physicians of it, but did not publish his results at the time.

The story shifts to Hartford, Connecticut, and Horace Wells (1815-1848), a dentist interested in developing a painless method for extracting teeth. Seeing a demonstration of the anesthetic properties of nitrous oxide in 1844, he had the gas administered to himself and parted with one of his teeth in painless fashion. Wells arranged to demonstrate his method before the surgeons of Massachusetts General Hospital, but apparently he removed the apparatus too soon; the patient awoke in pain; and the dentist left in disgrace.

Wells's debacle was witnessed by William T. G. Morton (1819-1868), who was both a dentist and a student in the Harvard Medical College. Pursuing the matter, Morton was led to ether by Charles T. Jackson (1805-1880), a physician and chemist of Boston. Experimenting first with animals and then on himself, Morton became satisfied that ether was both anesthetic and safe. In some manner he induced Dr. John Collins Warren (1778-1856), a leading surgeon of Boston, to try the agent in an operation on October 16, 1846. The operation was unflawed, and a month later the first paper on ether "anesthesia" appeared (the word was suggested by Oliver Wendell Holmes). Within a year surgeons all over the world had employed the new procedure.

The combination of efficient anesthesia and antisepsis opened new specialties in thoracic, cardiovascular, abdominal, and neural surgery. It also produced the zealous phase described previously as often following major scientific discoveries. Disease conditions for which no accepted procedure existed were now open to a surgical approach. A number of false starts would have to occur before the optimal operation could be devised for, say, removal of the stomach or gallbladder. But the twin obstacles to surgical progress that had existed for all of history were effectively overcome within the third quarter of the nineteenth century.

The Limits of Therapy

No one would dispute the fact that inhabitants of industrialized societies are healthier now than at any time in recorded history. More of us live longer, and the lives we live are freer of disease than Vesalius, Harvey, or Pasteur could ever have dreamed.
The conventional wisdom holds that our unprecedented good
health is due to the personal intervention of physicians equipped
with unprecedented understanding of the human body in health
and disease, which has been the theme of our story to this point.
The careful reader will already be troubled by any such simple,
straightforward interpretation of the available facts. In the section on specific prevention, it was pointed out that mortality
from the most important infectious diseases was waning before
specific remedies were available to physicians and patients.
Excepting smallpox, the same can be said of specific immunizations. Thomas McKeown, who has prepared the most searching
analysis of the role of personal physician intervention in all this,
concluded:

> If I were St. Peter admitting to heaven on the basis of achievement on
> earth, I would accept on proof of identity the accident surgeons, the den-
> tists, and with a few doubts, the obstetricians; all, it should be noted in
> passing, dealing mainly with healthy people. The rest I would refer to
> some celestial equivalent of Ellis Island, for close and prolonged inspec-
> tion of their credentials.[15]

McKeown's reading of recent history is that it was not the
work of personal physicians which controlled the contagious diseases, but improvements in nutrition, hygiene, and birth control.
Unlike others dealing with similar historical data, such as Ivan
Illich, McKeown would not dismantle the entire health care system, but finds a useful role for personal physicians and medical
investigators.

If his data are accurate, it is difficult to find serious fault with
the major thrust of McKeown's analysis. The available statistics
on morbidity and mortality, imperfect though they are, do dictate the conclusion that many of the important contagious diseases were diminishing before physicians had specific preventives or cures. Still, it should be kept in mind that the statistics of

disease do not reflect the healer's entire function. The qualitative aspects of life must be counted as well as the quantitative.

Mortality and morbidity figures on pneumonia reveal how many persons contract the disease and recover in a given period. McKeown maintains that the effect of chemotherapy on pneumonia mortality was not significant for the period he studied. But what of the person who contracted pneumococcal pneumonia before antibiotics and did not die? In a typical case the extreme distress of high fever and agonizing pain lasted between seven and ten days. For the fortunate who survived the initial attack without suffering such complications as lung abscess, pericarditis, meningitis, or endocarditis, another week in bed, followed by a varying period of ambulatory convalescence, was the rule. By way of contrast, the pneumonia patient on effective antibiotic treatment often becomes afebrile and comfortable within twenty-four hours; complications are relatively rare, and the period of disability is greatly reduced. And it must be remembered that pneumococcal pneumonia is an extremely common human disease.

There is a lengthy list of conditions for which the ministrations of individual physicians have directly improved the quality of life. Before penicillin the child who recovered from scarlet fever was too often left deaf and mute. Those who survived other streptococcal infections developed rheumatic heart disease or chronic kidney failure. The babies of untreated syphilitic mothers, if they survived, suffered bone deformities, hydrocephalus, mental retardation, blindness, and deafness. Before gonococcal mothers were treated with penicillin and their newborn babies with silver nitrate, many of these children were blinded by gonococcal ophthalmia. A fractured hip in an elderly person formerly meant permanent confinement in bed, permanent, that is, until a visitation by pneumonia, "the old person's friend." Today the hip is pinned or the entire joint replaced. Sufferers of hypothyroidism formerly passed a lifetime of torpidity, at times misdiagnosed as mental retardation. Today, on thyroid hormonal replacement, they frequently return to a normal existence. The same can be said of those who suffer deficient or excessive production of hormones manufactured by the pituitary, adrenal, parathyroid, ovaries, and other glands. In all of these conditions and a host of others, patients who survived in the nineteenth century faced periods of debilitation that could last fifty years or more. The emotional and economic drain on the family was immense, and if the victim was the breadwinner, the family might literally be destroyed.

Finally there is the matter of reassurance. Suffering is not limited to illness but results as well from fear of illness and death. A great deal of suffering is alleviated daily by nothing more than the physician's reassurance that the current pain or bleeding or dizziness does not mean serious illness or death. And that reassurance can only be effective if given by one who is trained to determine when disease is not present as well as when it is.

None of what has been said in the preceding is intended as a commentary on the adequacy of the present health care system in the United States. Nor is it meant as an apology for the current heavy use of drugs and diagnostic procedures. The point has been only to suggest that preventive and therapeutic agents applied by personal physicians have had salutary effects not reflected in naked statistics on mortality. Without taking exception to McKeown's conclusions on the importance of diet, hygiene, and birth control, it is suggested that specific prevention and specific therapy have also played a significant role in the management of disease in the broadest sense. Beyond that it is likely that the role of the individual physician in preventing mortality itself will assume greater importance when the last half of the twentieth century is fully assessed.

Notes

1. Quoted by Ludovici, L. J. *Fleming: Discoverer of Penicillin.* London: Andrew Dakers, 1952, p. 154.

2. Halsband, R. *The Life of Lady Mary Wortley Montagu.* Oxford: Clarendon Press, 1956, p. 71.

3. Osler, W. "Recent Advances in Medicine," *Science* 17:170, 1891.

4. Shaw, B. *Selected Plays with Prefaces.* New York: Dodd, Mead, & Company, 1948, vol. 1, p. 10.

5. Temkin, O., quoting Leoniceno in *The Double Face of Janus and Other Essays in the History of Medicine.* Baltimore: Johns Hopkins University Press, 1977, p. 454.

6. Joseph, H. *Shakespeare's Son-in-Law: John Hall, Man and Physician.* Hamden, Conn.: Archon Books, 1964, pp. 12, 25.

7. Holmes, O. W. *Currents and Counter-Currents in Medical Science.* Boston: Ticknor and Fields, 1861, p. 38.

8. Olmsted, J.M.D. *François Magendie.* New York: Schuman's, 1944, p. 157.

9. Berman, A. "The Heroic Approach in Nineteenth Century Therapeutics," *Bull. Am. Soc. Hosp. Pharm.* 11:322, 1954.

10. Holmes, *Currents and Counter-Currents,* pp. 38–39.

11. King, L. S. *A History of Medicine: Selected Readings.* Baltimore: Penguin Books, 1971, pp. 157–158.

12. Dowling, H. F. *Fighting Infection: Conquests of the Twentieth Century.* Cambridge: Harvard University Press, 1977, p. 93.

13. Paget, S. *John Hunter.* London: T. Fisher Unwin, 1907, p. 27.

14. Brown, J. *Rab and His Friends.* London: J. M. Dent & Sons, 1934, p. 42.

15. McKeown, T. *The Role of Medicine: Dream, Mirage, or Nemesis?* London: Nuffield Provincial Hospitals Trust, 1976, p. x.

Bibliographic Commentary

My overview of therapeutics derives principally from two works by E. H. Ackerknecht, "Aspects of the History of Therapeutics," *Bull. Hist. Med.* 36:389–419, 1962, and *Therapeutics from the Primitives to the Twentieth Century,* New York: Hafner Press, 1973. Other useful general essays include C. Keele, "One Hundred Years of Progress in the Drug Treatment of Disease," *Roy. Soc. Health J.* 83:325–330, 1963; O. Temkin, "Historical Aspects of Drug Therapy," in P. Talalay, *Drugs in Our Society,* Baltimore: Johns Hopkins University Press, 1964; L. S. King, "The Road to Scientific Therapy," *J. Am. Med. Assn.* 197:250–256, 1966; and C. D. Leake, *An Historical Account of Pharmacology to the Twentieth Century,* Springfield, Ill.: Charles C. Thomas, 1975.

Comments on the philosophy of therapy draw heavily on O. Temkin, *The Double Face of Janus,* Baltimore: Johns Hopkins University Press, 1977, pp. 472–484.

The best single article on therapeutic excesses in the nineteenth century is by A. Berman, "The Heroic Approach in Nineteenth-Century Therapeutics," in J. W. Leavitt and R. L. Numbers, *Sickness and Health in America,* Madison: University of Wisconsin Press, 1978. A useful series of essays covering a wide variety of subjects is by M. J. Vogel and C. E. Rosenberg, *The Therapeutic Revolution,* Philadelphia: University of Pennsylvania Press, 1979.

The rationale for bloodletting has been analyzed in great detail by P. H. Niebyl in *Venesection and the Concept of the Foreign Body,* Ph.D. diss., Ann Arbor: University Microfilms, 1970, and in more limited aspects in his "The Helmontian Thorn," *Bull. Hist. Med.* 45: 570–595, 1971.

The decline of bloodletting in America is discussed by L. S. Bryan, Jr., "Bloodletting in American Medicine, 1830–1892," *Bull. Hist. Med.* 38:516–529, 1964, and the story for England is related by P. H. Niebyl, "The English Bloodletting Revolution, or Modern Medicine Before 1850," *Bull. Hist. Med.* 51:464–483, 1977.

Excerpts in English from the relevant work by Pierre Louis are found as "Researches on the Effects of Blood-Letting, 1836" in L. King, *A History of Medicine: Selected Readings,* Middlesex, England: Penguin Books, 1971. For an excellent account of the persistence of bloodletting, see G. B. Risse, "The Renaissance of Bloodletting: A Chapter in Modern Therapeutics," *J. Hist. Med. and Allied Sciences* 34:3-22, 1979.

The reasons for the American decline of heroic therapy generally have been studied by R. H. Shryock, *The Development of Modern Medicine*, Madison: University of Wisconsin Press, 1979; Charles Rosenberg in *The Therapeutic Revolution* (see above); Rosenberg, "The Practice of Medicine in New York a Century Ago," in *Sickness and Health in America* (see above); and especially, Rosenberg, *The Cholera Years*, Chicago: University of Chicago Press, 1962; and finally, W. G. Rothstein, *American Physicians in the Nineteenth Century*, Baltimore: Johns Hopkins University Press, 1972.

The story of Withering and digitalis draws on F. W. Peck and K. D. Wilkinson, *William Withering of Birmingham*, Baltimore: Williams and Wilkins Co., 1950, and A. R. Cushny, "William Withering," in Z. Cope, ed., *Sidelights on the History of Medicine*, London: Butterworth and Co., 1957.

Excerpts from *Lind's Treatise on the Scurvy* appear in L. S. King, *A History of Medicine* (see above), and selected references to the disease have been compiled by A. L. Bloomfield, *A Bibliography of Internal Medicine: Selected Diseases*, Chicago: University of Chicago Press, 1960.

Ehrlich's story derives from I. Galdston, *Behind the Sulfa Drugs*, New York: D. Appleton-Century Company, 1943; L. G. Stevenson, "Antibacterial and Antibiotic Concepts in Early Bacteriological Studies and in Ehrlich's Chemotherapy," in I. Galdston, ed., *The Impact of the Antibiotics on Medicine and Society*, New York: International Universities Press, 1958; and H. F. Dowling, *Fighting Infection: Conquests of the Twentieth Century*, Cambridge: Harvard University Press, 1977, which also tells the story of Domagk. Also of real value is J. Parascandola, ed., *The History of Antibiotics. A Symposium*. Madison, Wisconsin: American Institute of History of Pharmacy, 1980.

The biography of Fleming by L. J. Ludovici, *Fleming: Discoverer of Penicillin*, London: Andrew Dakers, 1952, is more objective, though not so elegantly written, as that by A. Maurois, *The Life of Sir Alexander Fleming*, New York: E. P. Dutton & Co., 1959. (See also Dowling, above.) H. W. Florey's contemporary account is found in "The Use of Micro-organisms for Therapeutic Purposes," *Brit. Med. J.* 2:635-642, 1945, and a recent biography is that by G. Macfarlane, *Howard Florey: The Making of a Great Scientist*, Oxford: Oxford University Press, 1979.

The history of clinical experimentation has been recounted by J. P. Bull, "The Historical Development of Clinical Therapeutic Trials," *J. Chronic Diseases* 10:218-248, 1959; F.H.K. Green, "The Clinical Evaluation of Remedies," in B. Lush, ed., *Concepts of Medicine*, New York: Pergamon Press, 1961; H. F. Dowling, "The Emergence of the Cooperative Clinical Trial," *Trans. Studies Coll. of Physicians, Philadelphia* 43:20-29, 1975; A. M. Lilienfeld, "*Ceteris Paribus:* The Evolution of the Clinical Trial," *Bull. Hist. Med.* 56:1-18, 1982; and A. M. Harvey, *Science at the Bedside*, Baltimore: Johns Hopkins University Press, 1981.

For the conceptual development of surgery, see L. M. Zimmerman and I. Veith, *Great Ideas in the History of Surgery*, New York: Dover Publications, 1967. Our improved understanding of the relationship between surgery and the

Church derives from D. W. Amundsen, "Medieval Canon Law on Medical and Surgical Practice by the Clergy," *Bull. Hist. Med.* 52:22–44, 1978. The crucial story of eighteenth-century French surgery is told by T. Gelfand, *Professionalizing Modern Medicine,* Westport, Conn.: Greenwood Press, 1980.

Hunter's work on aneurysms is described by E. Home, "An Account of Mr. Hunter's method of performing the operation for the cure of Popliteal Aneurism," in J. E. Erichsen, *Observations on Aneurism,* London: The Sydenham Society, 1844.

There are innumerable accounts of the development of general anesthesia. My version follows C. D. Leake, "The Historical Development of Surgical Anesthesia," *Scientific Monthly* 20:304–328, 1925; T. E. Keys, *The History of Surgical Anesthesia,* New York: Dover Publications, 1963; and J. D. Trent, "Surgical Anesthesia, 1846–1946," in G. H. Brieger, ed., *Theory and Practice in American Medicine,* New York: Science History Publications, 1976.

McKeown's thesis was developed in two principal books, T. M. McKeown, *The Modern Rise of Population,* New York: Academic Press, 1976, and *The Role of Medicine,* London: Nuffield Provincial Hospitals Trust, 1976. See also J. Powles, "On the Limitations of Modern Medicine," *Sci., Med., and Man* 1:1–30, 1973.

11
HEALTH, DISEASE, AND ILLNESS

"There's a classical Tay-Sachs in 219C," is a remark which would not convey much to the uninitiated, but which would be perfectly clear to the health professional in training on a pediatrics ward. Translated to useful English the sentence would read, "There is a child in room 219C who suffers a genetic disease marked by severe mental deterioration, blindness, and death before the age of four." When he speaks of the "Tay-Sachs in 219C," the health professional unwittingly echoes an essential contradiction that has characterized medical theory and practice for more than two thousand years. Is there really a disease, a discrete entity, inhabiting the unfortunate child in 219C? Is it proper to speak of diseases as things having an actual reality, a natural history of their own? The ontologists in the history of disease would say yes. "Surgery does the ideal thing," wrote a popular health columnist of the 1930s; "it separates the patient from his disease. It puts the patient back to bed and the disease in a bottle."[1]

But is the person whose kidney stone has just been put in a bottle really "separated from his disease?" When he leaves the operating room he takes with him the same pathologic physiology that produced the kidney stone initially, an infection such as tuberculosis, any of a number of metabolic disorders, or the same personal habits which may contribute to a certain percentage of kidney stones whose origin remains obscure. Somehow it seems inadequate to view disease as a thing apart from the individual in whom it takes place. And so it has seemed to the anti-ontologists, those who view disease as a unique process in time in a single individual, as what we might term illness as distinct from disease. The contradiction is that the study of disease demands thinking in generalizations, but the practice of medicine deals with sick individuals. Tay-Sachs the disease is a generic abstraction applied to a constellation of signs, symptoms, and pathological findings. But Tay-Sachs the illness is a unique process in one individual. It may or may not have all the stigmata of Tay-Sachs the disease, but even if it does, it remains unique because the human vessel in which the dismal process unfolds is itself unique.

The question of disease vis-à-vis illness is not simply a philosophical plaything, though medical savants have had a fine (and often frustrating) time toying with it. Whether society and its health professionals are disease- or illness-oriented has vital implications for the patient. A predominantly disease-oriented medical person tends toward cookbook medicine. The disease is something apart from the patient, an invader of sorts. As soon as this physician can assign a diagnostic term to his patient, the next actions are more or less automatic. If the blood pressure is 175/95 and no specific cause can be found, the label is essential hypertension, and one action is salt restriction. Never mind that the patient is eighty-two years old and his principal remaining joy is his daily visit to the festive board.

The opposite conceptual extreme has hazards of a different sort. The physician who is inordinately illness-oriented has the merit of approaching his patients holistically, but if he is ignorant of disease, may miss the diagnosis and, for example, operate needlessly or too late.

Further, physicians today, as always, have experienced a profound need to clarify their conception of disease. Whatever the theory, whenever the time, wherever the place, medical men have striven to define precisely which human ailments are to be defined as disease. The task has never been as simple as one might imagine.

Distinguishing between disease and illness is attractive

because of its simplicity. It can also be confusing, because the two words are commonly used as synonyms. The matter is complicated further because many terms have been used to denote the two concepts. In the discussion that follows, these will be generally disregarded in favor of the terms ontological and physiological. Ontological will be used to describe disease as an independent entity with a natural history of its own. Physiological (biographical, historical) will mean the story of disease in an individual patient.

Even reduced to the two basic conceptions of ontological and physiological, the story remains extremely complex. Indeed, a full treatment would fill several volumes and more than exhaust the patience of the casual student of the history of disease. Some sort of summary treatment must be attempted, but in so doing, the reader must continually remind himself that many details are being omitted, that a few opinions have been selected to reflect the dominant view of a given time, and that a full treatment would reveal a much more complicated story. So warned, we may turn to an overview of the ontological and physiological conceptions as they played off against one another in the history of disease.

Ancient Concepts

Concepts of disease in ancient Egypt, Israel, and Mesopotamia were too diffuse and vague to fit easily into either the ontological or the physiological compartment. Disease was a punishment, whether for an unwitting violation of taboo or a deliberate offense against the gods or men. At the same time there was no formal or rational attempt to exclude natural elements of disease causation. A few anatomic relationships were understood, such as the connection between the heart beat and arterial pulse, and a network of blood vessels was postulated through which disease could spread to various parts of the body. Earlier we saw that a number of useful approaches to the management of disease were developed among ancient Hebrews and Egyptians even as the primary conceptual framework remained religious and magical.

Given the general outlook of the ancient Greeks, it is not surprising that they took a holistic view of man and his diseases.

Neither is it surprising to find philosophers taking an active role
in such speculations. Plato needed no firsthand experience to
perceive the logical pitfalls in compartmentalizing human illness. In *Charmides* he wrote that if a disease of the eyes is to be
cured the entire body must be treated, and that a common error
among contemporary physicians was that they separated body
and soul.

The school of Greek medical thought most congenial to
modern physicians began in the fifth century B.C. and, as noted,
is associated with the name of Hippocrates. It will be recalled
that for Hippocratic physicians disease was natural and thus susceptible to profitable study. Indeed, it was their repeated careful
clinical observations that brought them to the ontological-
physiological dichotomy. They were less troubled by the problem than it appears they should have been. Their close study of
sick persons inevitably led Hippocratic physicians to the notion
of specific diseases. The same set of symptoms was encountered
time and again and even permitted a reasonable prediction of the
outcome of a given case. At times they even applied names to
these symptom complexes, such as pleurisy and pneumonia. At
the same time they left no doubt of their physiological orientation. Disease was a process in time. Diseases were characterized
by rhythms described variously as acute, chronic, exacerbation,
relapse, return, intermission, resolution, acme, paroxysm, crisis,
and convalescence. These rhythms at times permitted more
accurate prognosis, an art the Hippocratics held in high esteem.
In *Acute Diseases,* as one example, we read that "in a bilious
fever, jaundice coming on with rigor before the seventh day car-
ries off the fever, but if it occur without the fever, and not at the
proper time, it is a fatal symptom."[2]

If the Hippocratics were so finely attuned to the differences in
individual sickness, how did they explain the similarities that
suggested the existence of specific diseases? The answer is that
they did not feel any compulsion to choose one idea and deny the
other. Diseases have their nature, but so do men. The manifestations of a given episode of disease will be colored, even determined, by the unique makeup of the patient. Thus it is important
not just to know the disease, but to assess the symptoms as determined by the nature of the individual. One works not with the

red and yellow that make up the mixture, but the orange that results.

As Greek medical thought spread first to Alexandria and then Rome, the two main approaches persisted. In Alexandria the ontological idea was championed by Erasistratus, who wrote books on paralysis, gout, and dropsy. In the second century A.D. the pendulum returned to Hippocratic doctrine due largely to Galen, who said in paraphrase, "A disease is not only a change of the body but also a change of this particular body." This means, for example, that in the treatment of epilepsy the physician not only must tailor the drugs to the patient's unique needs, but vary the entire regimen as the body changes day by day. After the decline of Rome, the Hippocratic-Galenic emphasis on the physiological approach to disease survived in the Greek-speaking East. There it was picked up by the Arabs and returned to the Latin West beginning in the eleventh century.

From Paracelsus to Sydenham

Still, the ontological idea was not entirely obscured. In the ninth century Rhazes gave us a glimpse of the revival of interest in generalizing diseases when he distinguished between smallpox and measles. The first significant break with Galenism generally and the physiological conception of disease in particular would not be made until Paracelsus in the sixteenth century. For Paracelsus there were as many specific diseases as "pears, apples, nuts and medlars," which is to say the number of diseases equals the number of objects that are not directly a part of man. Diseases then are specific and arise outside the body. Such convictions made Paracelsus a prime ontologist and influenced our next principal, the physician and chemist Johannes van Helmont. For van Helmont disease "is due to a creative 'seed' which gets hold of a part of the material frame of the body and 'organises' it according to its own schedule of life." As with Paracelsus, we may spare ourselves the details and conclude that for van Helmont it is the disease, not the patient, which varies. To that extent van Helmont's conception was distinctly ontological.[3]

In addition to their intrinsic importance, Paracelsus and van Helmont are significant because they illustrate the gathering momentum of an ontological movement which in some minds reached its peak with Thomas Sydenham, the "arch-ontologist," as he has been described, of the seventeenth century. But a subtle distinction enters at this point. In general Sydenham was less interested in classification than in discovering types. Thus he could write that the same symptoms one "would observe in the sickness of a Socrates you would observe in the sickness of a simpleton," in the same way that if one "should accurately describe the colour, the taste, the smell, the figure, etc., of one single violet," one would find that it essentially described "all the violets of that particular species upon the face of the earth."[4]

The attempt to divide diseases into species and genera goes back at least as far as ancient Greece. For Sydenham this process, and even more important, the nature of the treatment to be employed, was to be based on experience at the bedside. In this he differed with his contemporary Thomas Willis (1622–1675) and the school of thought which looked to the basic sciences and the laboratory approach for a rational way of understanding and treating disease. Beginning in 1666 Sydenham published a series of works containing detailed descriptions of smallpox, dysentery, syphilis, measles (which he distinguished from scarlatina), and gout, his personal nemesis from the age of thirty on. His aim was to lead physicians away from theorization divorced from clinical experience and back to the bedside study of disease. Later he would be dubbed "the English Hippocrates," and indeed he thought of himself as a Hippocratist, but, for our purposes, he was anything but. The Hippocratic writers described individual illnesses, not diseases. For them, as noted, each episode of illness was a unique event which could never happen again. Sydenham, on the other hand, was describing typical syndromes which he knew from past experience and which he would recognize when he encountered them again. In short, diseases were entities, and his view was ontological. Still, the record does not permit the contrast to be drawn strictly in terms of black and white. The Hippocratics, as we have already seen, particularly in the Cnidian treatises, were involved in distinguishing individual diseases as well. The difference was one of emphasis.

The Iatromechanists

The laboratories and theorizations from which Sydenham wished to extricate medical thinking were largely those of chemistry and physics. The lead pursued by Willis had begun with Paracelsus, followed by van Helmont, who emphasized the importance of chemistry in human biology. This doctrine was extended in the seventeenth century by the Leyden clinician Franz de le Boë, or Sylvius (1614–1672) as he is usually called, and by Willis. For Sylvius the final products of the body's physiological processes were acids and alkalis. If these agents existed in balance, health was the result. If the body's equilibrium was upset, "acrimoniae" were produced. These could be either acidic or alkaline, and once in the blood they produced disease. Treatment was aimed at restoring the physiologic balance.

Sylvius became the principal spokesman of the physician-chemists, or iatrochemists as they came to be called. Humoral pathology was not destined to disappear quickly, but the iatrochemists represented another crack in the wall. They retained elements of humoralism – the unitary conception of disease and the notion of health as balance – but the ephemeral humors were now replaced by substances that could be seen and manipulated in the laboratory as well as in the body. Whether or not the iatrochemists perceived the situation as such, humoral pathology was straining to accommodate the new chemistry of the seventeenth century.

Four years before Sylvius died, the man was born who would become the leading exponent of another school of medical thought, the iatrophysicists. This was Giorgio Baglivi (1668–1707), a physician who grew up in southern Europe under the influence of Galileo and his fellow physicists and mathematicians. René Descartes (1596–1650) had proclaimed the human body a machine controlled by mechanical laws. Baglivi carried this notion to its logical extreme. The teeth became scissors, the blood vessels a collection of tubes, and the lungs a set of bellows. The basic problem with the iatromechanical doctrines was that they contributed little that was useful to medical practice. Baglivi, for example, simply refused to allow his clinical practices to be dictated by his theories. Indeed, at the bedside his skills and accomplishments led him to be termed the Italian Sydenham. Anatomy and chemistry were important to medical practice, true, but not an end in themselves, as the iatrophysicists and iatrochemists would have it. In part that is why Sydenham, whose nosology was not all that influential in the seventeenth century, emerged as more influential in the perceptions of medical men in the eighteenth.

The Rise of Nosology

The first significant attempt to put into concrete form Sydenham's suggestion that diseases be arranged in much the way that botanists classified plants was made by François Boissier de Sauvages (1706-1767). In 1769 was published his *Nosologia methodica*. In it Sauvages divided diseases into ten classes which were subdivided into forty orders, thence to genera and finally to species, of which he discerned no fewer than 2,400. His earlier attempts at classifying diseases had been crude and unsuccessful. *Nosologia methodica* was a more learned effort, even though it was flawed by the fact that Sauvages was not identifying 2,400 diseases; for the most part what he was describing were symptoms. Still, the model had wide appeal. Before the end of the eighteenth century similar attempts were made in Edinburgh, Dublin, Vienna, and Lyons. Only the first of these, that published in 1769 by William Cullen (1712-1790), was any improvement on Sauvages.

As has been observed, the eighteenth-century nosologists did not improve on Sydenham in any significant way. Sydenham had attempted to characterize specific diseases by their symptoms and natural courses. The nosologists created no new clinical entities, but rather grouped and regrouped all the symptoms and syndromes already known to Sydenham. Their books nonetheless had great influence on medical practice in the eighteenth century. For all their complexity, they appeared to simplify the management of illness. The physician had only to identify the disease by its symptoms and place it in the nosological scheme, and the proper treatment was forthcoming. There was a further attraction in rigid classification; the practice of medicine was possible without resort to any of the contending theories of disease causation and mechanism that followed one another with confusing rapidity during the eighteenth century.

The Century of Medical Systems

Sauvages, unlike most of his eighteenth-century contemporaries, could be comfortable without a wholly developed theory of disease causation. He was satisfied with the belief that the causes of disease could never be appreciated by the physician's senses. Others were busily constructing the successive theoretical edifices that were to identify the eighteenth century as the century of great medical systems. Only the more successful of these can be presented here in abbreviated form, in an attempt to capture something of the conceptual flavor of the time.

For Friedrich Hoffmann (1660–1742), the body was akin to a hydraulic machine, with its activity determined by a vague nervous fluid. The fluid was secreted by the brain and carried throughout the body by the nerves and blood. Acute diseases generally resulted from an excess of nervous fluid, which produced spasm. Chronic diseases came about when the fluid was diminished, producing lack of bodily tone. Treatment was by opposites, using antispasmodics or stimulants as the diagnosis indicated.

Another influential systematist was William Cullen, a nosologist whose 1769 book, as noted, had the merit of reducing Sauvages's encyclopedia of signs and symptoms into groups, which we would call syndromes. Cullen, who happened to believe that muscles were continuations of nerves, taught that disease was largely a matter of nervous disorder. He is further representative of the great theoretical architects of the eighteenth century in that he rose to dominate his medical scene only to be assessed later as having not added one important fact to the science of medicine.

Cullen's pupil, the "disputatious and disreputable" John Brown (1735–1788), extended Cullen's ideas and arrived at a medical system that had great vogue in Germany, Italy, and the United States. To Brown life was nonexistent unless external stimuli were acting on an organized body. If the stimuli were too strong, excitement resulted, producing sthenic diseases. If too weak, excitation was lowered and asthenic diseases resulted. The appeal lay in its simplicity as applied at the bedside. The physician had only three matters to determine. Was the disease general or local, sthenic or asthenic, and to what degree? Treatment followed more or less automatically and consisted of two principal agents, alcohol and, above all, opium. Brown's system was a model of neatness and simplicity and attracted wide notice in the third quarter of the eighteenth century and afterwards.

The man who serves best as an example of systematization in the United States is Benjamin Rush (1745-1813). In part as a result of his experiences in the 1793 yellow fever epidemic in Philadelphia, Rush came to believe that all fevers had a single exciting cause, an "irregular action or convulsion" of the blood vessels. In the end he extended his convictions on the unitary nature of fever to disease in general. All diseases were due to spasms of the arteries. In another example of the dictum that the conception of disease tends to dictate the remedial actions taken, Rush extended the heroic purging and bleeding he had used to combat yellow fever until it became the central regimen of his medical practice at large.

Though their systems did not long survive them, Hoffmann, Cullen, Brown, Rush, and the other systematizers of the eighteenth century form an important link in our story. First, theirs were the dominant conceptual forces of the eighteenth century. Second, they demonstrate that medicine must have a theoretical basis if it is to claim professional status in its own eyes, as well as those of the public. Third, they show the persistence of at least two elements of the older humoral pathology they strove to replace—disease as a result of imbalance and all disease originating in a single basic cause. Finally, they are significant for what they meant to the events that followed. In the nineteenth century disease would be defined in terms of deviation from the normal, that is, by numerical data. Such a definition depends on a physiological basis for disease. Physiological functions vary within a range called normality, and when the variation is too great, disease results. Though he was capable of no real precision in measuring the strength of his stimuli or their effects on the body, Brown and those around him were employing the principle of deviation from the normal in their use of the sthenic-asthenic tension.

The Nineteenth Century

In the French Clinical School of the first half of the nineteenth century, ontologists and physiologists contended head to head. It was here, it may be remembered, that Corvisart and Laennec were applying the new tools of physical diagnosis to make some sense of diseases of the heart and lungs. In such a setting one might imagine the ontologists would dominate, but in the end it was the physiologists who held the upper hand.

High among the ontologists was Pierre Bretonneau (1771–1852), who spent his medical life not in the ferment of Paris but as a provincial in Tours. Bretonneau was particularly impressed by the specific appearance of lesions of the skin and mucous membranes. With his 1826 publication on diphtheria, it can be said that the "scientific history" of that disease began. He also demonstrated typhoid's characteristic lesions of the intestinal mucosa and was convinced that on such specific evidence the diagnosis, prognosis, and treatment depended. Bretonneau's influence was not as powerful as it might have been under other circumstances. As noted, his work was not in the center of the French medical stage. Further, he was not heavily disposed to committing his ideas and conclusions to writing. And finally, he was overshadowed by a far more forceful personality, François Broussais (1772–1838), who had a totally different idea of the nature of disease.

Broussais, as had Brown, adopted the notion that life depended on external and internal stimuli or irritation. In disease, certain organs became excessively or pathologically stimulated. Such stimulation (irritation) was localized and produced inflammatory changes that were visible as anatomical lesions. These lesions were to be viewed as disturbances of function, that is, of physiology, and focussed primarily in the stomach or intestine.

Thus for Broussais there were no specific diseases. Cancer and smallpox were merely inflammations, or the tracks left by inflammations. So inspiring was he that one of his students was moved to prove the nonexistence of a specific virus for syphilis.

To do so he inoculated himself with pus from a fresh syphilitic discharge. On schedule he developed a chancre, followed by generalized syphilis, and in a fit of depression he killed himself. To counteract the irritation Broussais developed what was termed "antiphlogistic" therapy. This involved a strict diet and the application of as many as fifty leeches, mostly on the abdomen. It was the system's popularity that led to the importation of millions of leeches into France at the time.

Broussais's localism was a step in the direction of understanding, but his physiology was largely of the armchair variety, having scant resemblance to the laboratory method already exploited by Magendie and soon to be taken to greater heights by Claude Bernard. In the end Broussais gave way to eclectics who leaned toward an anatomico-pathological orientation. Nevertheless, except for a few echoes of Sydenham in the German school of natural history around 1840, ontology, in the esteem of physicians, was all but dead between 1820 and 1880. Between 1865 and 1869 Villemin demonstrated that tuberculosis reproduces itself and cannot be reproduced other than by itself, in short that it was specific. But among his contemporaries it was not so perceived. Rather, tuberculosis was held to result from many different internal and external agents. In many minds the whole notion of specificity threatened to immobilize medical progress. If one subscribed to the notion that chronic diseases were specific, then research perforce would be limited to a search for specific remedies or preventives.

Disease as Deviation from the Normal

The ancient Greeks must be visited one last time. Plato in *Timaeus* put forth the idea that disease resulted from disharmony among the four humors, a conception traced earlier in these pages through the Hippocratic physicians and Galen. Put another way, disease in the humoral system was a deviation from the normal. Some have maintained that the Greeks saw disease and health in pure terms, that a person is either ill or well. There is, however, rather conclusive evidence of the concept of relative health in ancient Greece. This should not surprise us, because it conforms to the reality of the human condition. What needs emphasis, and what the Greek notion of relative health says to us, is that the concepts of illness and health are often defined by cultural factors that may at times pay little attention to the suffering or disability involved. In our society, women suffering dysmenorrhea usually may not assume the role of patient, with its attendant benefits and responsibilities. Similarly, a person may be all but prostrated by a common cold and still be expected to perform normally at work. This interpretation of the insignificance of the common cold is so pervasive that physicians shedding the virus in large numbers are expected to continue caring for patients in office and hospital even though the infection poses a serious threat to individuals who are ill from other conditions.

The problem of assessing normality in the tension between illness and health, then, is inherent in any theory of disease. But the problem has been perceived differently at different times. What was added in the nineteenth century was a greater emphasis on quantification, an attempt to circumscribe more definitively the limits of normality by the use of numbers. This is not to say that biological measurements had not been employed before. The Alexandrian Greeks had used a clepsydra, or water clock, to time the pulse. The ingenious seventeenth-century physician Santorio Santorio (1561–1636) devised a thermometer for determining body temperature and was even able to detect the body's loss of weight through insensible perspiration by weighing his own body, his intake of food and water, and his loss through excreta. Still, medicine was slow to accept the importance of biometrics in clinical practice. As late as 1860, C. A. Wunderlich (1815–1877), the man who is often credited with popularizing clinical thermometry, was still trying to convince his colleagues that the device was both practical and useful. It was not until 1871 that physicians of the Meath Hospital reported with apparent pride that temperatures were determined routinely twice daily in their institution.

The advent of better tools for measuring biological functions and the late nineteenth-century emphasis on hospital practice, in which physicians could accumulate large numbers of cases of the same disease, gave impetus to the notions of both specific pathological entities and of disease as a deviation from the normal. In addition the ontological cause was greatly abetted by the new bacteriology. Now it was no longer necessary to postulate some vague archaeus; the invading germs could be seen, grown, and injected into animals, each time producing the same pathological picture.

Once again the matter was not so simple. Typhoid Mary, as we saw, had a gallbladder full of pathogenic microorganisms, clearly a deviation from the normal. But she had no symptoms. Other obfuscating data accumulated. When amebiasis struck white persons in South Africa, few symptoms resulted. The middle-class Indians, infected by the same organisms, suffered diarrhea and minor intestinal trouble, but the Bantu developed liver abscesses. The same ameba, depending on racial and social factors, produced human reactions ranging from the negligible to death. Many such instances accumulated to indicate that the mere presence of a normally virulent germ could not be equated with disease. Perhaps it was impossible to draw a line between health and disease. Perhaps the definition of normality was a chimera in the world of biological reality.

Impediment

To get around the problem of the elusive limits of normality, physicians in the nineteenth century adopted the concept of impediment. In brief this stated that before a deviation from normal could be labeled disease, the patient had to exhibit some significant physical or social limitation. Actually it would be more accurate to say they *returned* to the concept of impediment, because this notion, too, can be traced back to antiquity. Galen defined health as a state in which there is neither pain nor impairment of normal functions.

As it developed there were problems with the concept of impediment as well. The normal limits of blood pressure are usually given as 140 systolic and 90 diastolic, but many persons carry a consistent reading of 150/95 with no symptoms and no limitation of social function. On the other hand there is the cardiac neurotic, whose father died suddenly of a heart attack at the age of forty-two. The complete range of physical and laboratory tests have been repeatedly normal, yet he refuses to budge out of his rocking chair. He is clearly restricted in his function, yet even if a pathologist could examine him cell by cell, no specific anatomical or physiological abnormality would turn up. In a working sense we might say that the hypersensitive stoic is diseased but not ill and the cardiac neurotic ill but not diseased. But this does not carry us very far toward an ideal definition of normality or disease.

Functional Disease

This already turbid stream was further muddied by what came to be termed functional disease, a concept that continues to perplex aspiring health professionals. In 1956 a medical student reported offering a free beer to any of his classmates who would compose a written definition of the term functional, "as used in the expression 'a functional disease' or 'a functional disorder.' " It seems that in class one day the professor had spoken of functional disease, and the student, in all innocence, had asked for an amplification of the term. Afterwards he was accused by his classmates of seeking attention by asking about something he already understood. The student denied any such wrongdoing and went on to express doubts as to whether his classmates understood the term even yet. Thus the offer of the free beer. Sixty-six students capitalized on this generosity. As the author suspected, the written definitions were scarcely characterized by uniformity. If one were to attempt a single composite definition embracing the major differences in the responses, it would run something as follows. Functional disease is idiopathic (cause unknown), psychogenic, or due to multiple causes and at times may be only a normal variation; it is sometimes, always, and never organic, and it is usually harmless, although it may result in death.

The perplexity is understandable because the term functional disease has taken on more than one meaning. In an earlier section we saw how the concept of functional disease came into nineteenth-century thinking when Adolf Kussmaul realized that the gastric contents he was extracting in the treatment of an acutely dilated stomach might reveal important information about the function of that organ. This innovation, it will be recalled, was generalized by Ottomar Rosenbach, applied to other organs, and came to signify a disease state wherein at times the function of an organ could be upset but without the presence of any changes the pathologist would label as disease.

Confusion set in when it became clear that purely mental activities could produce abnormalities in the function of an organ. Worry, for example, increases the flow of hydrochloric acid in the stomach. As time passed, for some, functional disease meant only that no organic lesion was demonstrable, for others that the disrupted function was psychogenic in origin, and for still others varying mixtures of the two.

Summary

It should be clear by this point that both the ontological and physiological concepts of disease have strengths and weaknesses. Aside from bacteria and demonic possession, the ontologist has difficulty in defining precisely what it is that causes disease. Even bacteria are troublesome in this regard, because, in theory at least, there should be a specific disease to match each type and strain of pathogenic microorganism, but this is not the case. Similarly, a deficiency of vitamin E can exist in human beings and not produce any as yet recognizable disease. The physiologist, on the other hand, has to stretch his tenets when he encounters case after case of measles or smallpox in which the course varies only infinitesimally.

As emphasized at the outset, the concept of disease is more than a matter of semantic nitpicking. A one-sided reliance on either ontology or physiology has significant implications for the practitioner as well as the academic, the investigator, and society. Lord Cohen, who favored the idea of disease as deviation from the normal, found five dangers in ontology.

(1) . . . It promotes a penny-in-the-slot machine approach to diagnosis by seeking for pathognomonic signs, especially the short cuts of the laboratory or instrument; (2) . . . it suggests that diagnosis is arrived at by comparing an unknown with a catalogue of knowns: the method of recognizing an elephant by having seen one before; (3) . . . it reduces thought to a minimum; (4) . . . it is of little help and may be positively misleading where the disease process varies significantly from the usual; and

(5) . . . it leads to all those dangers associated with a label which Cowper implied when he wrote of those — "who to the fascination of a name, Surrender judgment, hoodwinked."[5]

A resolute rejection of all ontological thinking poses problems as well. Students entering the study of medicine learn about disease by the use of names. They hold tuberculous lungs in their hands and view cancerous cells under a microscope. It is difficult to imagine anyone learning the essentials of useful pathology without giving names to diseases. Further, in medical practice there is something to be said for recognizing an elephant by having seen one before. In dermatology, for example, the process is extremely common, and it is doubtful that replacing it with a greater physiological orientation would serve either physician or patient, at least in the present state of the art. Finally, the use of ontological constructs has had unquestionable value in campaigns to eradicate disease by preventive means. It is impossible to imagine the worldwide campaigns against smallpox or malaria or mounting a March of Dimes to eradicate poliomyelitis without thinking in terms of disease entities.

Neither the ontological nor the physiological outlook is essentially wrong. What is required is a balanced outlook, an ability to think in terms of specific disease at one time and individual illness at the other. The "Compleat Physician," if such an ideal existed, would know the basic science and clinical manifestations of tuberculosis, but he would also be sensitive to the unique personal, family, and social ramifications of tuberculosis in a particular person. He would understand not just the tissue reaction to the tubercle bacillus, which is similar in all cases, but the human reactions of all those affected by a specific instance of tuberculosis, and these vary from one illness to another.

Notes

1. Clendening, L. *Modern Methods of Treatment*. St. Louis: C. V. Mosby Company, 1931, p. 19.

2. Adams, F. *The Genuine Works of Hippocrates*. New York: William Wood and Company, 1886, vol. 1, p. 270.

3. Pagel, W. "Van Helmont's Concept of Disease — To Be or Not to Be? The Influence of Paracelsus," *Bull. Hist. Med.* 46:419–454, 1972.

4. Latham, R. G. *The Works of Thomas Sydenham*. London: The Sydenham Society, 1848, p. 15.

5. Cohen, H. "The Evolution of the Concept of Disease," in Lush, B. *Concepts of Medicine*. New York: Pergamon Press, 1961, p. 168.

Bibliographic Commentary

The literature on the conception of disease is far too voluminous to allow for anything more than highly selective listing. Two most useful articles are by O. Temkin, "Health and Disease" and "The Scientific Approach to Disease: Specific Entity and Individual Sickness," which appear in *The Double Face of Janus*, Baltimore: Johns Hopkins University Press, 1977, pp. 419-440 and 441-455.

Other important works include L. King, *Medical Thinking*, Princeton N.J.: Princeton University Press, 1982; W. Riese, *The Conception of Disease*, New York: Philosophical Library, 1953; B. Lush, *Concepts of Medicine*, New York: Pergamon Press, 1961; L. J. Rather, "Towards a Philosophical Study of the Idea of Disease," in C. M. Brooks and P. F. Cranefield, eds., *The Historical Development of Physiological Thought*, New York: Hafner, 1959; R. H. Shryock, "The Interplay of Social and Internal Factors in the History of Modern Medicine," *Scientific Monthly* 76:221-230, 1953; and C. R. Burns, "Diseases Versus Healths: Some Legacies in the Philosophies of Modern Medical Science," in H. T. Engelhardt, Jr., and S. F. Spicker, eds., *Evaluation and Explanation in the Biomedical Sciences*, Dordrecht, Holland: D. Reidel Publishing Co., 1975; and two articles by C. Boorse, "On the Distinction Between Disease and Illness," *Phil. and Public Affairs* 5:49-68, 1975, and "Health as a Theoretical Concept," *Phil. Sci.* 44:542-573, 1977.

Recent analyses of this ancient problem include F. K. Taylor, *The Concepts of Illness, Disease and Morbus*, Cambridge: Cambridge University Press, 1979, and A. L. Caplan, H. T. Engelhardt, Jr., and J. J. McCartney, eds., *Concepts of Health and Disease*, Reading, Mass.: Addison-Wesley, 1981.

The Greek notion of relative health has been discussed by F. Kudlien, "The Old Greek Concept of 'Relative' Health," *J. Hist. Behav. Sci.* 9:53-59, 1973. Ancient examples of specific diseases are found in I. M. Lonie, "The Cnidian Treatises of the *Corpvs Hippocraticvm*," *Classical Quarterly*, n.s., 15:1-30, 1965. Galen's views on the subject are analyzed by O. Temkin, "Galenicals and Galenism in the History of Medicine," in I. Galdston, ed., *The Impact of the Antibiotics on Medicine*, New York: International Universities Press, 1958.

The title aptly describes the contribution by W. Pagel, "Van Helmont's Concept of Disease – To Be or Not to Be? The Influence of Paracelsus," *Bull. Hist. Med.* 46:419-454, 1972.

For some of the finer nuances of Sydenham's ideas about disease, which vary somewhat from traditional interpretations, see D. G. Bates, "Thomas Sydenham: The Development of His Thought, 1666-1676," Ph.D. diss., Johns Hopkins University, 1975.

L. S. King has produced three books which are invaluable with regard to medical thought in the seventeenth and eighteenth centuries: *The Road to Medical Enlightenment, 1650-1695*, New York: American Elsevier, 1970; *The Medical*

World of the Eighteenth Century, Chicago: University of Chicago Press, 1958; and *The Philosophy of Medicine: The Early Eighteenth Century,* Cambridge: Harvard University Press, 1978. For an excellent depiction of the head-to-head struggle between the systematists and their opponents, see G. B. Risse, "The Quest for Certainty in Medicine: John Brown's System of Medicine in France," *Bull. Hist. Med.* 45:1-12, 1971. The evolution of Rush's thinking is examined in C. Holmes, "Benjamin Rush and the Yellow Fever," *Bull. Hist. Med.* 40:246-263, 1966.

The starting point for the nineteenth century is K. Faber, *Nosography in Modern Internal Medicine,* New York: Paul B. Hoeber, 1923. Broussais's story is told by E. H. Ackerknecht, "Broussais, or A Forgotten Medical Revolution," *Bull. Hist. Med.* 27:320-343, 1953. Ideas of normality and impediment are discussed by R. P. Hudson, "The Concept of Disease," *Ann. Int. Med.* 65:595-601, 1966; C. D. King, "The Meaning of Normal," *Yale J. Biol. and Med.* 17:493-501, 1945; A. Kaplan, "A Philosophical Discussion of Normality," *Arch. Gen. Psychiat.* 17:325-330, 1967; and J. Ruesch and C. M. Brodsky, "The Concept of Social Disability," *Arch. Gen. Psychiat.* 19:394-403, 1968.

For the clinical utility of distinguishing between disease and illness, see A. R. Feinstein, *Clinical Judgment,* Baltimore: Williams and Wilkins, 1967. A call for a "new" biomedical model which sounds more like a return to Hippocratic thought is G. L. Engel, "The Need for a New Medical Model: A Challenge for Biomedicine," *Science* 196:129-136, 1977.

Mention was made in the text of the fact that yellow fever played a significant role in the thinking and action of Benjamin Rush concerning disease generally. The manner whereby diseases themselves have shaped medical thought has been seriously neglected historically. G. B. Risse has explored the subject in "Epidemics and Medicine: The Influence of Disease on Medical Thought and Practice," *Bull. Hist. Med.* 53:505-519, 1979. Earlier efforts in this regard include E. H. Ackerknecht, "Malaria in the Upper Mississippi Valley, 1760-1900," *Supplements to the Bull. Hist. Med.,* no. 4, Baltimore: Johns Hopkins University Press, 1945, and C. E. Rosenberg, *The Cholera Years: The United States in 1832, 1849 and 1866,* Chicago: University of Chicago Press, 1962.

APPENDIX: THE HIPPOCRATIC OATH

I swear by Apollo Physician and Asclepius and Hygieia and Panaceia and all the gods and goddesses, making them my witnesses, that I will fulfill according to my ability and judgment this oath and this covenant:

To hold him who has taught me this art as equal to my parents and to live my life in partnership with him, and if he is in need of money to give him a share of mine, and to regard his offspring as equal to my brothers in male lineage and to teach them this art – if they desire to learn it – without fee and covenant; to give a share of precepts and oral instruction and all other learning to my sons and to the sons of him who has instructed me and to pupils who have signed the covenant and have taken an oath according to the medical law, but to no one else.

I will apply dietetic measures for the benefit of the sick according to my ability and judgment; I will keep them from harm and injustice.

I will neither give a deadly drug to anybody if asked for it, nor will I make a suggestion to this effect. Similarly I will not give to a woman an abortive remedy. In purity and holiness I will guard my life and my art.

I will not use the knife, not even on sufferers from stone, but will withdraw in favor of such men as are engaged in this work.

Whatever houses I may visit, I will come for the benefit of the sick, remaining free of all intentional injustice, of all mischief and in particular of sexual relations with both female and male persons, be they free or slaves.

What I may see or hear in the course of the treatment or even outside of the treatment in regard to the life of men, which on no account one must spread abroad, I will keep to myself holding such things shameful to be spoken about.

If I fulfill this oath and do not violate it, may it be granted to me to enjoy life and art, being honored with fame among all men for all time to come; if I transgress it and swear falsely, may the opposite of all this be my lot.

INDEX

About the Author

Robert P. Hudson received his M.D. from the University of Kansas, where he is currently Chairman of the Department of the History and Philosophy of Medicine. He has written numerous articles which have appeared in prominent journals such as the *Journal of the American Medical Association, Annals of Internal Medicine, Journal of the Kansas Medical Society, Bulletin of History of Medicine,* and *Clio Medica.*